# Principles of Substance Abuse Prevention for
# Early Childhood
## A Research-Based Guide

# PRINCIPLES OF SUBSTANCE ABUSE PREVENTION
## FOR EARLY CHILDHOOD:
## A RESEARCH-BASED GUIDE

This publication is available for your use and may be reproduced **in its entirety** without permission from NIDA. Citation of the source is appreciated, using the following language:

Source: National Institute on Drug Abuse; National Institutes of Health; U.S. Department of Health and Human Services.

**March 2016**

# Table of Contents

Acknowledgements ................................................................................................................................ 1

Introduction ........................................................................................................................................... 3

Principles of Substance Abuse Prevention for Early Childhood ...................................................... 7

Principle 1 (Overarching Principle): Intervening early in childhood can alter the life course trajectory in a positive direction ..................................................................................................................... 7

Principle 2: Intervening early in childhood can both increase protective factors and reduce risk factors 7

Principle 3: Intervening early in childhood can have positive long-term effects ............................. 7

Principle 4: Intervening in early childhood can have effects on a wide array of behaviors ............ 7

Principle 5: Early childhood interventions can positively affect children's biological functioning ........... 8

Principle 6: Early childhood prevention interventions should target the proximal environments of the child .................................................................................................................................................. 8

Principle 7: Positively affecting a child's behavior through early intervention can elicit positive behaviors in adult caregivers and in other children, improving the overall social environment .............. 8

Chapter 1: Why is Early Childhood Important to Substance Abuse Prevention? ........................... 11

What does the life course perspective show about risk for drug abuse and how to prevent it? ........ 12

What are the major influences on a child's early development? ...................................................... 14

Chapter 2: Risk and Protective Factors ........................................................................................... 21

What are some important early childhood risk factors for later drug use? ..................................... 21

What if a child has multiple risk factors? ........................................................................................ 26

What are some important protective factors that can offset risk factors? ..................................... 28

Chapter 3: Intervening in Early Childhood ..................................................................................... 33

What contexts do early childhood interventions target? ................................................................ 37

Do early childhood interventions target all children or just those at highest risk? ....................... 38

What are some characteristic features of early childhood interventions? ...................................... 39

How does changing the behavior of parents and teachers help children? ..................................... 42

Who benefits the most from early childhood interventions? ......................................................... 42

Chapter 4: Research-Based Early Intervention Substance Abuse Prevention Programs .............. 47

Prenatal/Infancy and Toddlerhood (Ages 0 to 3 Years) ................................................................. 49

Universal Programs ..................................................................................................................... 49

Durham Connects .................................................................................................................... 49

Selective Programs ...................................................................................................................... 49

Early Steps, Family Check-Up (Early Steps FCU) ................................................................... 49

Family Spirit ............................................................................................................................. 50

Nurse Family Partnership ........................................................................................................ 51

Preschool (Ages 3 to 6 Years) ....................................................................................................................52

    Selective Programs.................................................................................................................................52

        Multidimensional Treatment Foster Care for Preschoolers (MTFC-P)....................................52

Transition to School (Ages 6 to 8 Years)...................................................................................................53

    Universal Programs ..............................................................................................................................53

        Caring School Community Program......................................................................................53

        Classroom-Centered (CC) Intervention................................................................................54

        Linking the Interests of Families and Teachers (LIFT). ....................................................55

        Raising Healthy Children (RHC). .........................................................................................56

        SAFEChildren...........................................................................................................................57

        Seattle Social Development Project (SSDP). ......................................................................58

    Selective Programs.................................................................................................................................59

        Early Risers "Skills for Success" Risk Prevention Program. ............................................59

        Kids in Transition to School (KITS)......................................................................................60

    Tiered Programs .....................................................................................................................................60

        Fast Track Prevention Trial for Conduct Problems. ...........................................................60

        Incredible Years® Parents, Teachers, and Children's Training Series...............................62

        Positive Action (PA). ..............................................................................................................63

        School and Homes in Partnership (SHIP)............................................................................64

Chapter 5: Selected Resources........................................................................................................................69

Appendix 1: From Theory to Outcomes—Designing Evidence-Based Interventions ...........................79

    Intervention Timing, Context, and Components................................................................................80

    Program Evaluation and Assessment of Benefit-Cost .....................................................................81

Appendix 2: Selecting and Implementing an Intervention .......................................................................85

    Determining Community Risk and Protective Factors......................................................................85

    Identifying the Target Population ........................................................................................................88

    Adapting Programs ................................................................................................................................89

    Collecting Data .......................................................................................................................................89

# Acknowledgments

This publication was written by Elizabeth B. Robertson, Ph.D., University of Alabama (formerly with the National Institute on Drug Abuse), Belinda E. Sims, Ph.D., National Institute on Drug Abuse, and Eve E. Reider, Ph.D., National Center for Complementary and Integrative Health. It was edited by Eric Wargo, Ph.D., National Institute on Drug Abuse. NIDA wishes to thank the following individuals for their guidance and comments during the development and review of this publication:

**Karl G. Hill, Ph.D.**
University of Washington

**Nicholas S. Ialongo, Ph.D.**
Johns Hopkins University

**Leslie Leve, Ph.D.**
University of Oregon

**David L. Olds, Ph.D.**
University of Colorado

**Naomi Stotland, M.D.**
University of California, San Francisco

NIDA also would like to thank the Community Anti-Drug Coalitions of America (CADCA) for helping organize a focus group of community leaders in reviewing this publication and the following individuals who participated in the focus group:

**B.J. Boyd, Ph.D.**
Cherokee National Behavioral Health

**Velma Overman**
Starfish Family Services

**Tanya Roberts**
Families in Action, Inc.

**Heather Warner**
Strategic Planning Initiative for Families and Youth

NIDA wishes to thank the following individuals for their contributions to the development of this publication:

**Nona Lu, M.D.**
Vanderbilt University

**Marisa Pinchas, M.P.H.**
Children's Hospital Los Angeles

**Sarah D. Lynne Landsman, Ph.D.**
University of Florida

# Introduction

Substance abuse and addiction are preventable disorders that interfere with normal healthy functioning, contributing to physical and behavioral health problems, injuries, lost income and productivity, and family dysfunction. While substance use generally begins during the adolescent years, there are known biological, psychological, social, and environmental factors that contribute to the risk that begin accumulating as early as the prenatal period. This creates opportunities to intervene very early in an individual's life and thereby prevent substance use disorders—and, along with them, a range of other related behavioral problems—long before they would normally manifest themselves.

The second edition of NIDA's *Preventing Drug Abuse Among Children and Adolescents* (2003) noted that "early intervention can prevent many adolescent risks." This special supplement to that volume reflects a growing body of research that has continued to accumulate showing that providing a stable home environment, adequate nutrition, physical and cognitive stimulation, warm supportive parenting, and good classroom management in the early years of a child's life (prenatal through age 8) can lead the child to develop strong self-regulation (i.e., emotional and behavioral control) and other qualities that protect against a multitude of risks and increase the likelihood of positive developmental outcomes. Positive effects of these interventions include delayed initiation and decreased use of drugs when the child reaches adolescence.

By adolescence, children's attitudes, behaviors, family interactions, and relationships—factors that may influence propensity to try or become addicted to drugs—are well established and not as easily changed. For young children already exhibiting serious risk factors for later drug use, delaying intervention until later childhood or adolescence may make it more difficult to overcome accumulated risk factors and achieve positive outcomes.

Our increased understanding of brain development and neuroplasticity across the first two decades of life also supports implementing early intervention. The prenatal, child, and adolescent brain is undergoing rapid and significant change, including the formation of new synapses and, after about age 5, the progressive pruning of unused synaptic connections and reinforcement of major circuits. Synaptic plasticity makes early childhood extremely sensitive to experiences and environmental influences (including family interactions and social contexts) that may act either as risk factors for later drug use and related problems or that may be protective against those risks. Thus the earlier an intervention occurs, the greater the potential to take advantage of biological, emotional, and behavioral sensitive periods to alter the course of development in a positive, healthy direction.

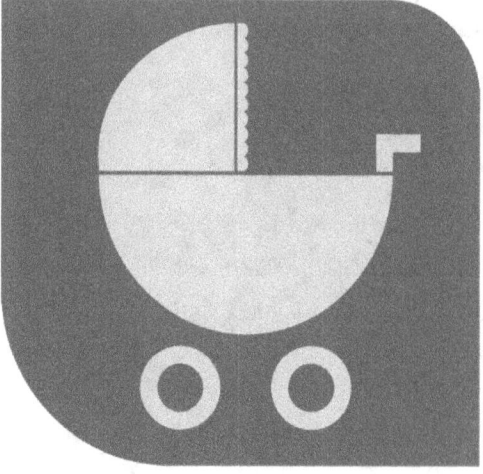

Research supports the value of interventions that reduce risk factors, promote protective factors, and increase access to resources (e.g., school- and community-based family support services) in the lives of young children and those closest to them. Substantial data from many long-term studies now indicate that intervening with children and families who are showing early risk factors for substance abuse is effective, and the benefits of such interventions continue into adolescence and young adulthood and even into adulthood.

Research has also found that a large number of early risk factors for substance abuse are simultaneously risk factors for other mental, emotional, and behavior problems. For example, early-onset externalizing behavior problems, such as aggressive and disruptive behaviors in the preschool years, have been found to relate to increased risk for outcomes such as conduct disorders, substance use, delinquency, and risky sexual behaviors in adolescence. Given that this is the case, it is not surprising that interventions designed to prevent substance abuse have shown many positive benefits that extend to other outcomes—including improved personal, social, and familial functioning; higher academic and career achievement; and less involvement with the juvenile justice system and mental health services.

Early childhood prevention interventions can be costly to implement, but the research balancing the benefits of these programs against their costs shows they are good—occasionally very good—investments. Among interventions for which such data are available, savings range from $2.88 for every dollar invested (the Nurse-Family Partnership, described in Research-Based Early Intervention Substance Abuse Prevention Programs) to as much as $25.92 (the Good Behavior Game, used in the Classroom-Centered Intervention) (Aos et al., 2004). Thus, a well-conceived and well-implemented intervention for very young children can not only dramatically improve the quality of life for the children and families involved but also benefit the community and society as a whole.

This guide, intended for parents, practitioners, and policymakers, begins with a list of 7 principles addressing the specific ways in which early interventions can have positive effects on development; these principles reflect findings on the influence of intervening early with vulnerable populations on the course of child development and on common elements of successful early childhood programs. This is followed, in "Why is Early Childhood Important to Substance Abuse Prevention?" and "Risk and Protective Factors," with an overview of child development from the prenatal period through age 8 (the span covered by this resource) and the various factors that either place a child at risk for later substance use or offer protection against that risk.

"Intervening in Early Childhood" describes common elements of early childhood interventions that target individual, family, school, and community precursors of drug use, abuse, and addiction. "Research-Based Early Intervention Substance Abuse Prevention Programs" includes information on specific early childhood intervention programs for which the National Institute on Drug Abuse (NIDA) has provided research support, and a section on "Selected Resources" provides links to many Federal agencies, professional and academic organizations, and non-governmental agencies that engage in early-childhood-prevention–related initiatives. Two appendices for policymakers, researchers, and practitioners go into greater detail on how early childhood interventions are designed and how to select the right intervention for a community's specific needs.

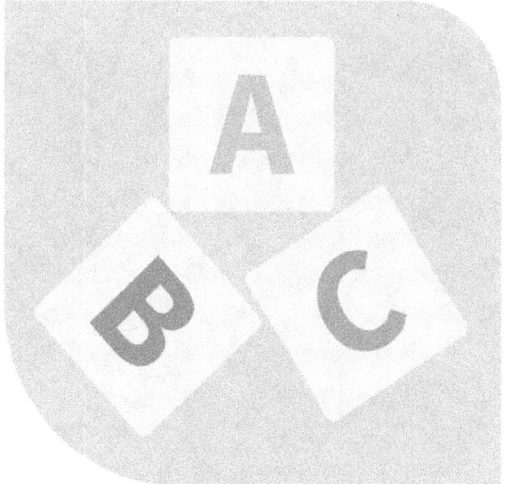

The "Selected References" include up-to-date sources that provide more in-depth coverage of all of the concepts, principles, and programs discussed.

Early childhood risks can lead to immediate and long-term problems that increase a child's chances of substance abuse and other problems in adolescence and later in life. It is now known that intervening early is a worthwhile strategy for setting children on a healthier path that may avoid these difficulties. NIDA hopes that this guide is helpful to substance abuse prevention efforts for children at home, in schools, and in communities nationwide.

## Selected Reference

Aos S, Lieb R, Mayfield J, Miller M, Pennucci A. Benefits and costs of prevention and early intervention programs for youth. Olympia, WA: Washington State Institute for Public Policy; 2004. Document No. 04-07-3901. http://www.wsipp.wa.gov/ReportFile/881/Wsipp_Benefits-and-Costs-of-Prevention-and-Early-Intervention-Programs-for-Youth_Summary-Report.pdf. Published September 17, 2004. Accessed February 3, 2015.

# Principles of Substance Abuse Prevention for Early Childhood

Seven principles of prevention for early childhood (which is defined here as the prenatal period and infancy through the transition to elementary school around age 8) have emerged from research studies funded (in full or in part) by NIDA. The detailed rationale for these principles appears in "Why is Early Childhood Important to Substance Abuse Prevention?," "Risk and Protective Factors," and "Intervening in Early Childhood."

Principle 1 (Overarching Principle): Intervening early in childhood can alter the life course trajectory in a positive direction (Kellam et al., 2008; Kitzman et al., 2010). Substance abuse and other problem behaviors that manifest during adolescence have their roots in the developmental changes that occur earlier—as far back as the prenatal period. While prevention can be effective at any age, it can have particularly strong effects when applied early in a person's life, when development is most easily shaped and the child's life is most easily set on a positive course.

*The following specific principles collectively provide support for Principle 1.*

Principle 2: Intervening early in childhood can both increase protective factors and reduce risk factors (August et al., 2003; Catalano et al., 2003). Risk factors are qualities of children and their environments that place children at greater risk of later behavioral problems such as substance abuse; protective factors are qualities that promote successful coping and adaptation and thereby reduce those risks. All children have a mix of both. Interventions aim to shift the balance toward protective factors.

Principle 3: Intervening early in childhood can have positive long-term effects (Degarmo et al., 2009; Shaw et al., 2006). Early childhood interventions focus on settings and behaviors that may not appear relevant for adjustment later in childhood or in adolescence, but they help set the stage for positive self-regulation and other protective factors that ultimately reduce the risk of drug use.

Principle 4: Intervening in early childhood can have effects on a wide array of behaviors (Beets et al., 2009; Hawkins et al., 2008; Snyder et al., 2010), even behaviors not specifically targeted by the intervention (Hawkins et al., 1999; Kellam et al., 2014; Lonczak et al., 2002). Because behaviors (both positive and negative) are linked to each other, risk factors for substance use may simultaneously put a child at risk for other problems such as mental illness or difficulties at school. This is why intervening to prevent one undesirable outcome may have a broad effect, improving the child's life trajectory in multiple ways.

Principle 5: Early childhood interventions can positively affect children's biological functioning (Bruce et al., 2009; Fisher et al., 2007). The benefits of intervention are not limited to behavioral or psychological outcomes—research has shown they can also affect physical health. For example, one intervention for young children in the foster care system looked at cortisol level, a biological measure of the stress response. Over time, the stress response of children receiving the intervention showed better regulation and became similar to that of children in the general population.

Principle 6: Early childhood prevention interventions should target the proximal environments of the child (Tolan et al., 2004; Webster-Stratton et al., 2008). The family environment is the most important context across all periods of early child development, and thus parents are a major target of many early childhood interventions (Dishion et al., 2008; Fisher et al., 2011). But as a child grows older, he or she typically spends more and more time out of the home, perhaps attending day care, then attending preschool followed by elementary school (Beets et al., 2009; Conduct Problems Prevention Research Group, 1999; Hawkins et al., 1999; Ialongo et al., 1999; Snyder et al., 2010). Interventions for different age groups and targeting different types of problems should focus on the most relevant context(s)—the home, school, day care, or a combination.

Principle 7: Positively affecting a child's behavior through early intervention can elicit positive behaviors in adult caregivers and in other children, improving the overall social environment (Fisher & Stoolmiller, 2008; Shaw et al., 2009). Behavioral changes in children and the adults who interact with them can be mutually self-reinforcing. Improving the child's family or school environment can, over time, cause the child's social behavior to become more positive and healthy (or pro-social); this, in turn, can elicit more positive interactions with others and improve the social environment as a result.

## Selected References

August GJ, Lee SS, Bloomquist L, Realmuto GM, Hektner JM. Dissemination of an evidence-based prevention innovation for aggressive children living in culturally diverse, urban neighborhoods: the Early Risers effectiveness study. *Prev Sci.* 2003;4(4):271-286.

Beets MW, Flay BR, Vuchinich S, et al. Use of a social and character development program to prevent substance use, violent behaviors, and sexual activity among elementary-school students in Hawaii. *Am J Public Health* 2009;99(8):1438-1445.

Bruce J, McDermott J, Fisher P, Fox N. Using behavioral and electrophysiological measures to assess the effects of a preventive intervention: a preliminary study with preschool-aged foster children. *Prev Sci.* 2009;10(2):129140.

Catalano RF, Mazza JJ, Harachi TW, Abbott RD, Haggrety KP, Fleming CB. Raising healthy children through enhancing social development in elementary school: results after 1.5 years. *J Sch Psychol.* 2003;41(2):143-164.

Conduct Problems Prevention Research Group. Initial impact of the Fast Track prevention trial for conduct problems: II. Classroom effects. *J Consult Clin Psychol.* 1999;67(5):648-657.

DeGarmo DS, Eddy JM, Reid JB, Fetrow RA. Evaluating mediators of the impact of the Linking the Interests of Families and Teachers (LIFT) multimodal preventive intervention on substance use initiation and growth across adolescence. *Prev Sci.* 2009;10(3):208-220.

Dishion TJ, Connell AM, Weaver CM, Shaw DS, Gardner F, Wilson MN. The Family Check-Up with high-risk indigent families: preventing problem behavior by increasing parents' positive behavior support in early childhood. *Child Dev.* 2008;79(5):1395-1414.

Fisher PA, Stoolmiller M, Gunnar MR, Burraston BO. Effects of a therapeutic intervention for foster preschoolers on diurnal cortisol activity. *Psychoneuroendocrinology.* 2007;32(8–10):892-905.

Fisher PA, Stoolmiller M, Mannering AM, Takahasi A, Chamberlain P. Foster placement disruptions associated with problem behavior: mitigating a threshold effect. *J Consult Clin Psychol.* 2011;79(4):481-487.

Fisher PA, Stoolmiller M. Intervention effects on foster parent stress: associations with child cortisol levels. *Dev Psychopathol.* 2008;20(3):1003-1021.

Hawkins JD, Catalano RF, Kosterman R, Abbott RD, Hill KG. Preventing adolescent health-risk behaviors by strengthening protection during childhood. *Arch Pediatr Adolesc Med.* 1999;153(3):226-234.

Hawkins JD, Kosterman R, Catalano R, Hill KG, Abbott RD. Effects of social development intervention in childhood 15 years later. *Arch Pediatr Adolesc Med.* 2008;162(12):1133-1141.

Ialongo NS, Werthamer L, Kellam SG, Brown CH, Wang S, Lin Y. Proximal impact of two first-grade preventive interventions on the early risk behaviors for later substance abuse, depression, and antisocial behavior. *Am J Community Psychol.* 1999;27(5):599-641.

Kellam SG, Brown CH, Poduska JM, et al. Effects of a universal classroom behavior management program in first and second grades on young adult behavioral, psychiatric, and social outcomes. *Drug Alcohol Depend.* 2008;95(Suppl 1):S5-S28.

Kellam SG, Wang W, Mackenzie ACL. The impact of the Good Behavior Game, a universal classroom-based preventive intervention in first and second grades, on high-risk sexual behaviors and drug abuse and dependence disorders into young adulthood. *Prev Sci.* 2014;15(Suppl. 1):S6-S18.

Kitzman H, Olds D, Cole R, et al. Enduring effects of prenatal and infancy home visiting by nurses on children: follow-up of a randomized trial among children at age 12 years. *Arch Pediatr Adolesc Med.* 2010;164(5):412-418.

Lonczak HS, Abbott RD, Hawkins JD, Kosterman R, Catalano RF. Effects of the Seattle Social Development Project on sexual behavior, pregnancy, birth, and sexually transmitted disease outcomes by age 21 years. *Arch Pediatr Adolesc Med.* 2002;156(5):438-447.

Shaw D, Connell A, Dishion T, Wilson M, Gardner F. Improvements in maternal depression as a mediator of intervention effects on early childhood problem behavior. *Dev Psychopathol.* 2009;21(2):417-439.

Shaw DS, Dishion TJ, Supplee L, Gardner F, Arnds K. Randomized trial of a family-centered approach to the prevention of early conduct problems: 2-year effects of the family check-up in early childhood. *J Consult Clin Psychol.* 2006;74(1):1-9.

Snyder FJ, Vuchinich S, Acock A, et al. Impact of the Positive Action program on school-level indicators of academic achievement, absenteeism, and disciplinary outcomes: a matched-pair, cluster randomized, controlled trial. *J Res Educ Eff.* 2010;3(1):26-55.

Tolan P, Gorman-Smith D, Henry D. Supporting families in a high-risk setting: proximal effects of the SAFEChildren preventive intervention. *J Consult Clin Psychol.* 2004;72(5):855-869.

Webster-Stratton C, Reid MJ, Stoolmiller M. Preventing conduct problems and improving school readiness: evaluation of the Incredible Years Teacher and Child Training Programs in high-risk schools. *J Child Psychol Psychiatry.* 2008;49(5):471-488.

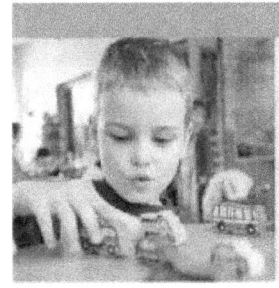

# Chapter 1
## Why Is Early Childhood Important to Substance Abuse Prevention?

Abundant research in psychology, human development, and other fields has shown that events and circumstances early in peoples' lives influence future decisions, life events, and life circumstances—or what is called the *life course trajectory*. People who use drugs typically begin doing so during adolescence or young adulthood (see "Adolescent Drug Use"), but the ground may be prepared for drug use much earlier, by circumstances and events that affect the child during the first several years of life and even before birth.

The first, overarching principle drawn from the research reviewed for this resource is that intervening early in childhood can alter the life course trajectory of children in a positive direction.

> *Principle 1: Intervening early in childhood can alter the life course trajectory in a positive direction.*

Early childhood, considered in this book to include the prenatal period through age 8, includes the following developmental periods:
- *Prenatal Period* (conception to birth)
- *Infancy and Toddlerhood* (birth to 3 years)
- *Preschool* (ages 3 through 6 years)
- *Transition to School* (ages 6 through 8 years)†

**Adolescent Drug Use**
Collection of data from the National Survey of Drug Use and Health (NSDUH) on age at first use of illegal drugs across the U.S. begins at age 12 years, with data from 2014 indicating that 3.4 percent of 12- to 13-year-old children have used an illegal drug in the past month (including inappropriate use of prescription drugs), 2.1 percent are current alcohol users, and 1.1 percent are current tobacco users (CBHSQ, 2015). In 2015, NIDA's annual Monitoring the Future (MTF) survey of adolescent drug use and attitudes showed that, by the time they are seniors, 64 percent of high school students have tried alcohol, almost half have taken an illegal drug, 31 percent have smoked a cigarette, and 18 percent have used a prescription drug for a nonmedical purpose (Johnston et al., 2016).

---

† The transition to school period is actually part of the middle childhood and early adolescence period (6 to 13 years) but is addressed separately in this book because it is a major and significant transition in the child's development. The middle childhood period is followed by adolescence (ages 13 to 18). The age range for the interventions that form the basis for the principles of prevention described in this resource is prenatal through 8 years.

The period of development covered in this guide is characterized by rapid orderly progressions of normal patterns of physical, cognitive, emotional, and social development. This development is marked by important *transitions* between developmental periods and the achievement of successive developmental *milestones* (see "Life Transitions" and "Developmental Milestones"). How successfully or unsuccessfully a child meets the demands and challenges arising from a given transition, and whether the child meets milestones on an appropriate schedule, can affect his or her future course of development, including risk for drug abuse or other mental, emotional, or behavioral problems during adolescence.

*The child's stage of life, aspects of his or her social and physical environments, and life events experienced over time all contribute to the child's physical, psychological, emotional, and cognitive development.*

A variety of factors, known as *risk factors*, can interrupt or interfere with unfolding developmental patterns in all of these periods and, especially, in the transitions between them. Prevention interventions designed specifically for early developmental periods can address these risk factors by building on existing strengths of the child and his or her parents (or other caregivers) and by providing skills (e.g., general parenting skills and specific skills like managing aggressive behavior), problem-solving strategies, and support in areas of the child's life that are underdeveloped or lacking.

Life events or transitions represent points during which the individual is in a period of change, and they are sometimes called sensitive, critical, or vulnerable periods (Brazelton, 1992; Bornstein, 1989). Although vulnerability can occur at many points along the life course, it tends to peak at critical life transitions, which present risks for substance abuse as well as opportunities for intervention. Thus transitions such as pregnancy, birth, or entering preschool or elementary school are prime opportunities to introduce skills, knowledge, and competencies to facilitate development during those transitions. Therefore, interventions are often designed to be implemented around periods of transition.

The life transitions diagram points to life course periods, contexts, and transitions or life events that together contribute to the development of the child from the prenatal period through young adulthood. (The life course continues through to the end of life, but this resource focuses on just the early years.)

## Life Transitions

Vulnerability to the risk factors for problems such as substance abuse can occur throughout the life course, but it tends to peak during critical life transitions. Transitions may be biological, such as puberty, or they may involve entering a new environmental context, such as attending school for the first time. How a child responds and adapts to these events is influenced by his or her cognitive, emotional, and social development at that point in time as well as past history, family relationships, and the surrounding world. Other transitions, such as parental divorce or military deployment of a parent, may not be predictably linked to a child's development, but these events or circumstances still require the child to adapt successfully (for instance to new people or new contexts). Because of their introduction of new potential risk factors, transitions are sometimes called sensitive, critical, or vulnerable periods, and they are prime opportunities for preventive intervention.

The figure below illustrates the development/life course trajectory from the prenatal period through young adulthood, indicating the periods of transition and life change that could represent both times of risk and periods where intervention could be of greatest benefit.

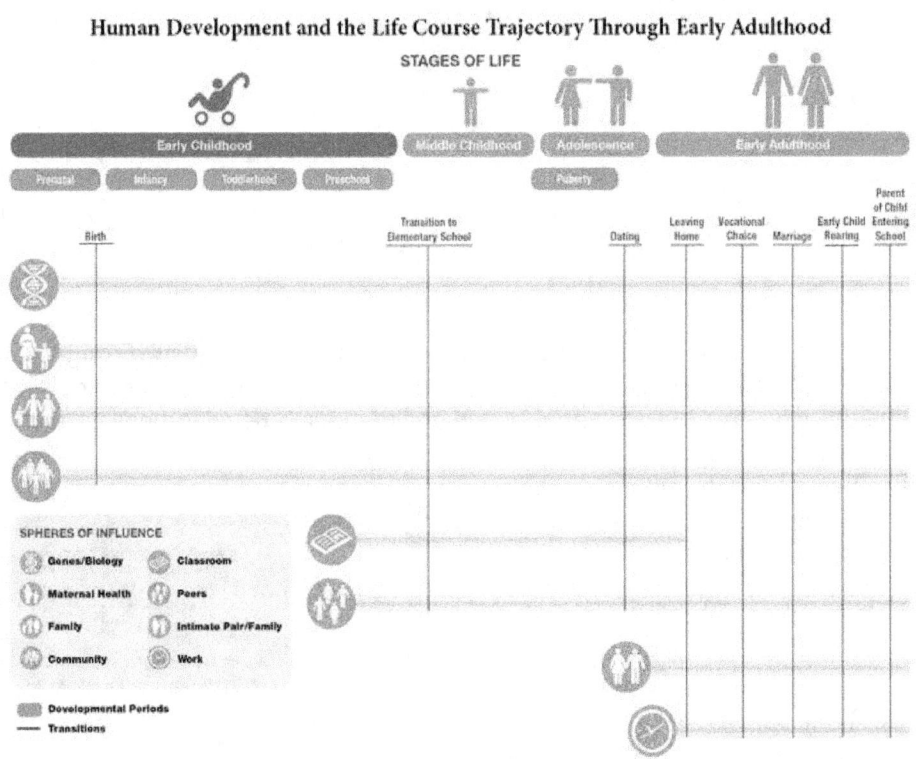

*Developmental periods, life course transitions, and contexts relevant to those transitions that contribute to the development of the child from the prenatal period through young adulthood (Kellam & Rebok, 1992).*

### Developmental Milestones

Developmental milestones refer to particular physical, cognitive, social, or emotional capabilities that are ordinarily acquired within a certain age range. For example, most infants crawl around 9 months and walk by 12 to 15 months; most toddlers can speak one- and two-word phrases between ages 1 and 2; and so on (see www.cdc.gov/ncbddd/actearly/milestones/index.html). Over the course of development, these emerging capabilities generally trigger changes in other people's expectations and responses—for instance, upon entering elementary school, teachers will expect children to be able to sit and be attentive. Achieving milestones within the expected time frame is an important signal that development is occurring in the expected manner and timeframe, and offers protection against risk factors for substance abuse and other problems later in development. Failure to achieve important milestones may indicate the need for early intervention.

This does not mean that a child who is well below average on a milestone will not eventually achieve that milestone (or will necessarily develop later problems); milestones can be achieved later in development, albeit with greater difficulty. Part of what makes it possible to achieve a milestone at a later time is the ability of the brain to change, adapt, and reorganize. This type of brain activity is called *plasticity*, and the brain remains plastic to some degree throughout life (Kellam & Rebok, 1992; Leighton et al., 1963; Weiss, 1949). However, very young children have the greatest neurological flexibility and potential for learning new skills and behaviors; brain structure stabilizes with age and it becomes increasingly difficult to alter (see "The Developing Brain, 0 to 8 Years").

## What are the major influences on a child's early development?

The changes unfolding throughout a child's development are influenced by a complex combination of factors. One of them is the *genes* the child inherits from his or her biological parents. Genetic factors play a substantial role in an individual's development through the course of life, influencing a person's abilities, personality, physical health, and vulnerability to risk factors for behavioral problems like substance abuse. But genes are only part of the story.

Another very important factor is the environment, or the *contexts* into which the child is born and in which the child grows up. The family/home environment is the context that most directly influences the young child's early development and socialization (see "Socialization"). This includes quality of parenting and other parenting influences such

### Socialization

Socialization refers to a process of acquiring and internalizing the behaviors, norms, and beliefs of the individual's society. It is a process that occurs across the course of development. During the early childhood period, both internal processes (such as learning style, attention, information processing) and the sum total of the child's social experiences in family, school, and community contexts affect socialization.

as genetic factors and family functioning. Also, siblings, if present, can influence a child's development and adjustment (e.g., internalizing and externalizing behaviors and substance use, as well as positive behaviors) (Dunn, 2005; Feinberg et al., 2013; Kramer & Conger, 2009; Pike et al., 2005). These influences may result from shared environmental experiences and interactions with parenting and other family factors (Burt et al., 2010; Neiderhiser et al., 2013). But conditions at home are also influenced by wider physical, social, economic, and historical realities—such as the family's socio-economic status and the affluence and safety (or lack thereof) of the community in which the family lives. As the child grows older and enters school, these wider environmental contexts influence him or her more directly.

What follows is an overview of the developmental influences and changes taking place during specific periods of early childhood development.

Prenatal Period

The genes, biological capacities, and innate temperament that children are born with inform the way they interact with the environment and people in it. Development is shaped by a combination of genetic and environmental factors (see "The Developing Brain, 0 to 8 Years.").

Even before a child is born, the context or environment plays an important role in development. It has long been known, for example, that if the mother smokes, drinks alcohol, or uses other drugs during her pregnancy, these substances can enter the body of the developing fetus and have significant effects on the development of the body and brain, and these effects may become risk factors for substance use later in the child's life (see "Risk and Protective Factors" for more information). There is also emerging evidence that both parents' past histories of substance use may affect their children via changes to gene expression (see "Epigenetics"). Also, poor nutrition during the prenatal period can have adverse effects on the development of the child's brain (National Research Council and Institute of Medicine, 2000; Prado & Dewey, 2014).

**Epigenetics**

Recent research in the emerging field of *epigenetics*, or the study of environmental influences on the way genes are expressed, suggests that both the mother's and father's past history of substance use, even before conception, may influence the health of their children. Studies in experimental animals have shown that substance use may cause changes in gene expression in a father's sperm and a mother's egg cells, which could then affect the growth and brain development of offspring, influencing their response to substances of abuse (Novikova et al., 2008; Vassoler et al., 2013; Szutorisz et al., 2014). Future studies will determine if this also occurs in humans.

## The Developing Brain, 0 to 8 Years

The brain is a dense network of nerve cells (neurons) and glial cells that support the neurons in various ways. The neurons are organized in circuits that control everything people think and do—from learning and movement to language, sensing, feeling, and exerting control over emotions and behaviors. The brain's development begins soon after conception, when cells in the embryo begin to form the basic structure of the central nervous system including the brain and spinal cord. How it develops is influenced by genetics, aspects of the environment such as nutrition and social interactions, and life experiences. The relative importance of these influences shifts over the course of life, and at any point they may interact in complex ways. For example, a particular genetic factor might impede the process of a child's language development; but if the child is born into a family where parents regularly talk or read to the child, it may foster language development and act to offset those genetic influences. Brain development is not simply the growth of new nerve cells and formation of synaptic connections (connections between neurons). Early in life, there is an overproduction of synaptic connections, and over the course of childhood and adolescence a process called *pruning* reduces the number of those connections. Connections that are used frequently become strengthened; those that are not are eliminated. For example, children are born with the capacity to understand and replicate sounds of all languages; however, over the course of development these abilities become specific to the language or languages to which they are exposed. Thus the neural connections that would allow further language development diminish in the middle childhood years.

Across childhood and adolescence, the cortex (the outer layer of the brain) matures at different speeds, as measured by its overall volume, its thickness, its surface area, and other characteristics that correspond to its functioning. Generally, areas at the back and sides of the brain that process sensory information (e.g., vision, hearing, and all types of body sensations) finish developing earliest, during childhood; frontal cortical areas, which handle emotional and behavioral control and other higher order executive functions, are the last to finish developing—only reaching maturity in early adulthood. Boys' and girls' brains differ in their pattern of brain maturation, with peak changes in cortical volume and surface area typically occurring later in boys (around age 10) than in girls (around age 8) (Raznahan et al., 2011).

The proportional genetic and environmental influences on various aspects of brain development are not the same across all brain regions. Recent twin studies have shown, for example, that variations in the thickness of the frontal cortex are more attributable to genetic factors than thickness of other areas of the cortex (Schmitt et al., 2014). Also, the relative influence of environmental and genetic factors in brain development shifts across the first three decades of life: The environment exerts its greatest proportional impact in early childhood and gradually lessens, relative to genetic influences, across later childhood and adolescence. This provides an important genetic and neurobiological rationale for intervening in early childhood, when changes in the individual's environment can have the greatest long-term impact.

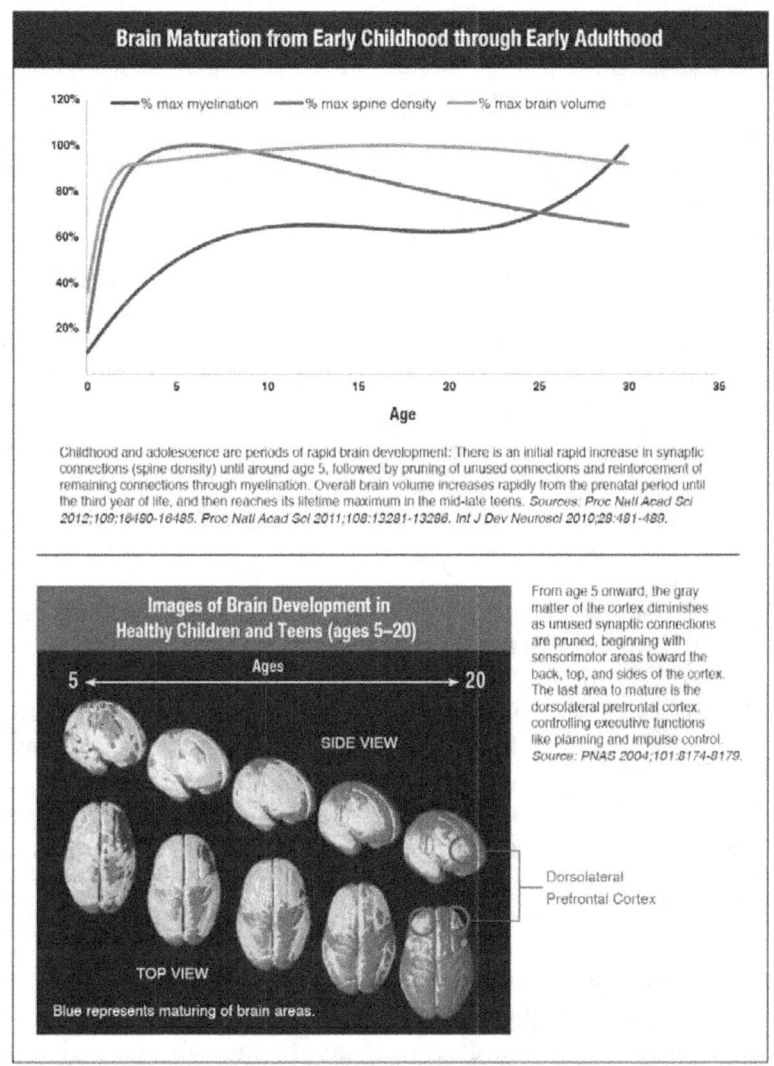

**Brain Maturation from Early Childhood through Early Adulthood**

— % max myelination   — % max spine density   — % max brain volume

Childhood and adolescence are periods of rapid brain development: There is an initial rapid increase in synaptic connections (spine density) until around age 5, followed by pruning of unused connections and reinforcement of remaining connections through myelination. Overall brain volume increases rapidly from the prenatal period until the third year of life, and then reaches its lifetime maximum in the mid-late teens. *Sources: Proc Natl Acad Sci 2012;109:16480-16485. Proc Natl Acad Sci 2011;108:13281-13286. Int J Dev Neurosci 2010;28:481-489.*

**Images of Brain Development in Healthy Children and Teens (ages 5–20)**

Ages
5 ← → 20

SIDE VIEW

TOP VIEW

Blue represents maturing of brain areas.

From age 5 onward, the gray matter of the cortex diminishes as unused synaptic connections are pruned, beginning with sensorimotor areas toward the back, top, and sides of the cortex. The last area to mature is the dorsolateral prefrontal cortex, controlling executive functions like planning and impulse control. *Source: PNAS 2004;101:8174-8179.*

Dorsolateral Prefrontal Cortex

## Infancy and Toddlerhood

Once the child is born, factors that contribute to the child's development include the quality of the nutrition and health care provided by the mother and other caregivers, the personality fit between infant and caregivers, and the ability of the caregivers to provide warmth and support. The child also plays a more active role in shaping his or her environmental context (see "Influence is not Just a One-Way Street").

**Influence is not Just a One-Way Street**
Within moments after birth, the infant's personality and overall health can influence the parent-child relationship and physical environment in significant ways. As the child grows older, his or her unfolding personality and needs influence the family environment, school environment, and wider social contexts, which in turn exert an influence on the child and others in the same surroundings.

Over the months following birth, the child adapts to and integrates into the surrounding world as he or she makes further developmental gains, including ongoing brain development. Through practice, the child ideally becomes proficient at basic skills using limited but growing sensory, motor, cognitive, and social capacities, meeting basic milestones along the way. As the infant learns to distinguish self from others, he or she instinctively focuses attention on the primary caregiver(s), usually parents.

For optimal positive development to occur, the primary caregiver(s) must consistently meet the child's needs, be nurturing, provide a predictable schedule, and provide developmentally appropriate stimulation. The closeness of the parent-child relationship during this early period provides a context for the child's development and his or her expectations about the world as well as for secure attachment to his or her caregiver(s). Secure attachment is one of the most crucial factors leading to healthy socialization and self-regulation, which are major protective factors against drug use and other behavioral problems.

Preschool

Throughout early childhood, even when the child enters preschool or attends day care, the family remains the most important context for development. Parents play a number of roles in the development of a young child's social, emotional, and cognitive competence, including establishing the structure and routines for parent-child interactions; maintaining a sensitive, warm, and responsive relationship style; and providing instructional practices and experiences that help the child acquire necessary developmental skills. Development of motor abilities and language skills are important in the preschool period, influencing the child's growing independence.

*Throughout early childhood, even when the child enters preschool or attends day care, the family remains the most important context for development.*

When a nurturing, responsive relationship does not exist, elevated levels of stress hormones can impede a child's healthy brain development (Debellis & Zisk, 2014; Thompson, 2014). Moreover, when a caregiver cannot provide attention and nurturing because of a history of trauma, chronic stress, and/or mental health problems, the child is more likely to develop behavioral, social, emotional, or cognitive problems (Madigan et al., 2012; Delker et al., 2014). Likewise, impaired judgment related to substance use can reduce a parent's ability to create a warm, supportive environment for the child (Barnard & McKeganey, 2004; Lam et al., 2007). Child abuse and neglect, social isolation due to illness or disability, and lack of constancy in the primary caregiver (as in the case of a child in institutionalized care) are also linked to growth (including brain growth and neuronal connectivity), cognitive, motor, social, and emotional problems (see for example, Behen et al., 2009; Martins et al., 2013; McCall, 2013; Koss et al., 2014). Many of the prevention interventions discussed in this guide are aimed at facilitating constant, nurturing, responsive caregiving to reduce risk and prevent child behavior problems.

## Transition to School

As the child grows older, new transitions and associated challenges occur. A major transition for young children is beginning elementary school. Even children who attended preschool or had been in day care can find the rules for behavior and academic requirements associated with elementary school difficult to adapt to and achieve. Readiness for school is something that occurs over time with experience and practice. Early intervention can help parents and schools assist children through this transition. Once in elementary school, teachers can help children to adjust by providing positive classroom management.

**Selected References**

Barnard M, McKeganey N. The impact of parental problem drug use on children: what is the problem and what can be done to help? *Addiction.* 2004;99(5):552-559.

Behen ME, Muzik O, Saporta AS, et al. Abnormal fronto-striatal connectivity in children with histories of early deprivation: a diffusion tensor imaging study. *Brain Imaging Behav.* 2009;3(3):292-297.

Bornstein, M.H. Sensitive periods in development: structural characteristics and causal interpretations. *Psychol Bull.* 1989;105(2):79-197.

Brazelton TB. *Touchpoints: The Essential Reference to Your Child's Emotional and Behavioral Development.* Reading, MA: Addison-Wesley Publishing Company; 1992.

Burt SA, McGue M, Iacono WG. Environmental contributions to the stability of antisocial behavior over time: are they shared or non-shared? *J Abnorm Child Psychol.* 2010;38:327-337.

Center for Behavioral Health Statistics and Quality (CBHSQ). *2014 National Survey on Drug Use and Health: Detailed Tables.* Rockville, MD: Substance Abuse and Mental Health Services Administration; 2015.

De Bellis MD, Zisk A. The biological effects of childhood trauma. *Child Adolesc Psychiatr Clin N Am.* 2014;23(2):185-222.

Delker BC, Noll LK, Kim HK, Fisher PA. Maternal abuse history and self-regulation difficulties in preadolescence. *Child Abuse Negl.* 2014;38(12):2033-2043.

Dunn J. Commentary: siblings in their families. *J Fam Psychol.* 2005;19(4):654-657.

Feinberg ME, Solmeyer AR, Hostetler ML, Sakuma KL, Jones D, McHale SM. Siblings are special: initial test of a new approach for preventing youth behavior problems. *J Adolesc Health.* 2013;53(2):166-173.

Johnston LD, O'Malley PM, Miech RA, Bachman JG, Schulenberg JE. *Monitoring the Future National Results on Drug Use: 1975-2015: Overview, Key Findings on Adolescent Drug Use.* Ann Arbor, MI: Institute for Social Research, The University of Michigan; 2016.

Kellam SG, Rebok GW. Building developmental and etiological theory through epidemiologically based preventive intervention trials. In: McCord J, Tremblay RE, eds. *Preventing Antisocial Behavior: Interventions from Birth through Adolescence.* New York, NY: Guilford Press; 1992:162-195.

Koss KJ, Hostinar CE, Donzella B, Gunnar MR. Social deprivation and the HPA axis in early development. *Psychoneuroendocrinology.* 2014;50:1-13.

Kramer L, Conger KJ. What we learn from our sisters and brothers: for better or for worse. In Kramer L, Conger KJ, eds. *Siblings as Agents of Socialization. New Directions for Child and Adolescent Development..* San Francisco, CA: Jossey-Bass; 2009, 126, 1-12.

Lam WK, Cance JD, Eke AN, Fishbein DH, Hawkins SR, Williams JC. Children of African-American mothers who use crack cocaine: parenting influences on youth substance use. *J Pediatr Psychol.* 2007;32(8):877-887.

Leighton DC, Harding JS, Macklin DB, Macmillan AM, Leighton AH. *The Character of Danger: Psychiatric Symptoms in Selected Communities.* Vol. 3. New York, NY: Basic Books; 1963.

Madigan S, Wade M, Plamondon A, Jenkins J. Maternal abuse history, postpartum depression, and parenting: links with preschoolers' internalizing problems. *Infant Ment Health J.* 2012;36(2):146-155.

Martins C, Belsky J, Marques S, et al. Diverse physical growth trajectories in institutionalized Portuguese children below age 3: relation to child, family, and institutional factors. *J Pediatr Psychol.* 2013;38(4):438-448.

McCall RB. The consequences of early institutionalization: can institutions be improved? - should they? *Child Adolesc Ment Health.* 2013;18(4).

National Research Council and Institute of Medicine. *From Neurons to Neighborhoods: The Science of Early Childhood Development.* Committee on Integrating the Science of Early Childhood Development. Jack P. Shonkoff and Deborah A. Phillips, eds. Board on Children, Youth, and Families, Commission on Behavioral and Social Sciences and Education. Washington, D.C.: National Academy Press; 2000.

Neiderhiser JM, Marceau K, Reiss D. Four factors for the initiation of substance use by young adulthood: a 10-year follow-up twin and sibling study of marital conflict, monitoring, siblings, and peers. *Dev Psychopathol.* 2013;25(1),133-149.

Novikova SI, He F, Bai J, Cutrufello NJ, Lidow MS, Undieh AS. Maternal cocaine administration in mice alters DNA methylation and gene expression in hippocampal neurons of neonatal and prepubertal offspring. *PLoS One.* 2008;3(4):e1919.

Pike A, Coldwell J, Dunn JF. Sibling relationships in early/middle childhood: links with individual adjustment. J Fam Psychol. 2005;19(4):523-532.

Prado EL, Dewey KG. Nutrition and brain development in early life. *Nutrition Review.* 2014;72(4):267-284.

Raznahan A, Shaw P, Lalonde F, et al. How does your cortex grow? *J Neurosci.* 2011;31(19):7174-7177.

Schmitt JE, Neale MC, Fassassi B, et al. The dynamic role of genetics on cortical patterning during childhood and adolescence. *PNAS.* 2014;111(18):6774-6779.

Szutorisz H, DiNieri JA, Sweet E, et al. Parental THC exposure leads to compulsive heroin-seeking and altered striatal synaptic plasticity in the subsequent generation. *Neuropsychopharmacology.* 2014;39(6):1315-1323.

Thompson RA. Stress and Child Development. *Future Child.* 2014 Spring;24(1): 41-59.

Vassoler FM, White SL, Schmidt HD, Sadri-Vakili G, Pierce RC. Epigenetic inheritance of a cocaine resistance phenotype. *Nat Neurosci.* 2013;16(1):42-47.

Weiss P. The biological basis of adaptation. In: Romano J, ed. *Adaptation.* Ithaca: NY: Cornell University Press; 1949:7-14.

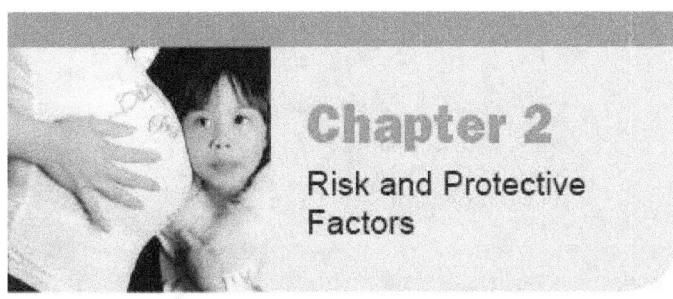

# Chapter 2
## Risk and Protective Factors

Research over the past three decades has identified many factors that can help differentiate individuals who are more likely to abuse drugs from those who are less likely to do so (Catalano et al., 2011; Hawkins et al., 1992). *Risk factors* are qualities of a child or his or her environment that can adversely affect the child's developmental trajectory and put the child at risk for later substance abuse or other behavioral problems. *Protective factors* are qualities of children and their environments that promote successful coping and adaptation to life situations and change. Protective factors are not simply the absence of risk factors; rather, they may reduce or lessen the negative impact of risk factors (Cowen & Work, 1988; Garmezy, 1985; Hawkins et al., 1992; Rutter, 1985; Werner, 1989).

*Principle 2: Intervening early in childhood can both increase protective factors and reduce risk factors.*

All children will have some mix of risk and protective factors. An important goal of prevention is to change the balance between these so that the effects of protective factors outweigh those of risk factors.

Both risk and protective factors may be *internal* to the child (such as genetic or personality traits or specific behaviors) or *external* (that is, arising from the child's environment or context), or they may come from the interaction between internal and external influences.

What are some important early childhood risk factors for later drug use?

Some factors that powerfully influence a child's risk for later substance abuse and other problems have their strongest effects during specific periods of development. Important examples include:

Prenatal Period
**Maternal smoking and drinking** can affect a developing fetus and may result in altered growth and physical development and cognitive impairments in the child (See "Pregnancy Matters: Use of Substances and Their Effects During Pregnancy").

**Pregnancy Matters: Use of Substances and Their Effects During Pregnancy**

Exposure to alcohol, tobacco, and other drugs of abuse during the prenatal period can affect children throughout their lifetime. Substances taken during pregnancy can cross the placenta, exposing the developing brain of the fetus to their effects. Examples of the effects of substance use during pregnancy include the following:

- **Smoking during pregnancy** has been linked to increased risk for slowed fetal growth and low birth weight, stillbirth, pre-term birth, infant mortality, Sudden Infant Death Syndrome, and respiratory problems.

- **Using alcohol during pregnancy** can cause miscarriage, stillbirth, and a range of lifelong disorders for the child known as Fetal Alcohol Spectrum Disorders (FASDs). FASDs can lead to physical, cognitive, and behavioral problems—for example, facial abnormalities; attention problems and hyperactive behavior; learning disabilities; poor reasoning and judgment skills; and problems with the heart, kidney, or bones.

- **The use of illicit drugs, such as cocaine, heroin, and marijuana, during pregnancy** can have a variety of adverse effects on children ranging from low birth weight to developmental problems related to behavior and cognition, such as impaired attention, problems with language development and learning, and behavior problems.

- **The use of some types of prescription drugs during pregnancy** may also have an impact on the child. Babies of mothers who chronically take opioid medications prescribed for pain or who are abusing those medications may be born with a physical dependency, causing withdrawal—a condition called Neonatal Abstinence Syndrome (NAS), which can require prolonged hospitalization of the infant and medication to treat.

The full extent of the consequences of substance use in pregnancy are not known because many confounding individual, family, and environmental factors such as nutritional status, extent of prenatal care, and socio-economic conditions make it difficult to determine the direct impact of prenatal substance use on the child. Therefore, abstinence is the best prevention.

<u>Infancy and Toddlerhood</u>

**Having a difficult temperament** in infancy may set the stage for the child having trouble with self-regulation later, as well as create challenges for the parent-child relationship (see "A Child's Temperament").

**Insecure attachment** during the child's first year of life can cause a child to be aggressive or withdrawn, fail to master school readiness skills, and have difficulty interacting with adults or other children (see "Attachment").

**Uncontrolled aggression** when a child is a toddler (2 to 3 years) can lead to problems when he or she enters preschool, such as being rejected by peers, being punished by teachers, and failing academically.

A Child's Temperament

All children are born with a unique temperament, or personality characteristics (Goldsmith et al., 1987) that make them easier or harder to care for. For example, babies who are easy to manage, adapt well to routines, and are responsive to parent care tend to elicit positive parenting behaviors, which will strengthen a growing, mutually satisfying parent-child relationship. On the other hand, some babies respond to their environment with arousal and distress; they may cry a lot, fuss when being changed and fed, and are not soothed by holding and rocking. These highly *reactive* infants are more likely to elicit parental frustration, impatience, and avoidance or neglect, which can potentially escalate into a pattern of negative family dynamics (Kochanska & Kim, 2013; Lee & Bates, 1985). These natural behavioral tendencies are the focus of early interventions for parents. Such interventions nurture appropriate expectations of infants by parents, strengthen positive parenting practices, and help parents to cope with frustrating situations.

<u>Preschool</u>

**Lack of school readiness skills** such as failure to have learned colors, numbers, and counting will put a child at a disadvantage in a classroom environment, setting the stage for poor academic achievement.

<u>Transition to School</u>

**Poor self-regulation** can lead to frustration and constant negative attention on the child by peers and teachers at school.

**Lack of classroom structure** in the school environment can lead to additional social and behavioral problems in children who have trouble switching from one activity to another.

Attachment

Attachment is the natural bond that develops between parent and child (Ainsworth et al., 1978; Bowlby, 1969; Bowlby, 1982). Usually this bond is positive and secure, but when children fail to develop secure attachments to their parents, they may perceive that the world is unsafe and eventually mistrust other people and distrust their own abilities to master the environment.

Attachment may be insecure due to particular experiences that get in the way of forming a secure bond, to specific personality characteristics of the parent and/or child, or to poor "fit" between characteristics of the parent and child. For example, an easy-going infant may react more calmly to a first-time parent's clumsy attempts at feeding, changing, and bathing him, whereas a more sensitive child might react with crying and other behaviors that could cause the parent to feel insecure about his or her capacity to parent. This in turn could affect interactions that promote attachment security (e.g., sensitive, contingent-responsive parenting). However, this is not deterministic. Good quality parenting is possible even when parent/child characteristics and experiences do not match up.

Early problems with attachment can lead to problems like acting out in school, poor academic achievement, and social isolation during the transition to elementary school (Fearon et al., 2010; Kochanska & Kim, 2012). Later on, during puberty, the transition to middle school, and adolescence, children with insecure attachment may associate with peers who exhibit problem behaviors and experiment with behaviors such as delinquency, substance use, and sexuality (Schindler & Bröning, 2015).

Any Developmental Period

Other risk factors can affect a child in any developmental period. Some important ones are:

**Stress** (Institute of Medicine and National Research Council, 2012; Masten, 1989; McEwen, 2010). All children experience stress at some point, and in fact a certain amount of stress helps young children develop skills for meeting challenges and coping with setbacks that inevitably occur in life. But chronic stressors like **family poverty** and stress that is intense or prolonged—such as **a parent's mental health problems** or a lingering **illness**—can diminish a child's ability to cope. These types of stress can even interfere with proper development, including brain development, and aspects of physical health like proper functioning of the immune system (Brown et al., 2009). This is particularly true of children who have experienced the extreme stress of **maltreatment**, such as abuse or neglect, by parents or caregivers (see "The Special Case of Abuse and Neglect"). Some children who experience a lot of stress early in life, even during the prenatal period, are more susceptible to the effects of later stressful life circumstances than other people (Raposa et al., 2014; Shonkoff et al., 2012; Turner & Lloyd, 2003).

**Parental substance use**: Parental substance use—including smoking, drinking, illicit drug use, and prescription drug abuse—can affect children both directly and indirectly. Substances used by a mother during pregnancy can cross the placenta and directly expose the fetus to drugs (see "Pregnancy Matters: Use of Substances and Their Effects During Pregnancy"), and substances can pass to a nursing infant through breast milk. When parents smoke in the home, it can also expose children to secondhand smoke, putting them at risk for health and behavioral problems (see "Secondhand Smoke"), as well as increasing children's likelihood of smoking when they grow older (Leonardi-Bee et al., 2011).

Parental substance use can also impact the family environment by giving rise to family conflict and poor parenting, which could increase risk for child abuse and neglect and involvement with the child welfare system (National Research Council and Institute of Medicine, 2009). Poor family functioning can increase the risk for multiple problem behaviors in children and adolescents, including risk for substance use and abuse

Secondhand Smoke
According to the surgeon general, there is no safe level of exposure to secondhand smoke (HHS, 2006). When children are exposed to it, they can develop the same kinds of health problems seen in smokers themselves. Secondhand smoke exposure in childhood is associated with upper and lower respiratory tract illnesses and asthma, as well as infection and tooth decay; it is the leading preventable cause of ear infection; and it is recognized as the most common preventable cause of Sudden Infant Death Syndrome (SIDS) (Zhou et al., 2014). Also, some components in secondhand smoke, such as carbon monoxide, are neurotoxic. Because children's brains are still developing, exposure to these chemicals can alter developmental trajectories and have long-lasting effects. Secondhand smoke exposure in children is linked to impaired executive brain function, which manifests most clearly as behavioral problems and an increased risk of ADHD (Pagani, 2014; Padrón et al, 2015).

(Aarons et al, 2008). Children with a family history of drug abuse also may have increased genetic risk for substance use (Kendler et al., 2003; Young et al., 2006), often manifested in combination with family or other environmental risk factors (Enoch, 2012). Children can learn about substance use from a very young age, especially if exposed to parental substance use and abuse (Noll et al, 1990). However, children are less likely to smoke, drink alcohol, or use other drugs when parents are clear that they do not want their children to do so, even if they use substances themselves (Jackson & Dickinson, 2006).

**Emergent mental illness.** Many mental illnesses have symptoms that can emerge during childhood and can increase risk for later drug abuse and related problems. For example, anxiety disorders and impulse-control disorders (such as ADHD) begin their onset prior to 11 years of age, on average (Kessler et al., 2005), but frequently symptoms may appear in early childhood. Symptoms associated with impulse-control disorders, such as aggressive disruptive behavior, as well as those associated with affective and psychotic disorders all increase the risk of substance use disorders and related problems in adolescence (Maslowsky et al, 2014; Gregg et al., 2007). (See "Drug Abuse and Mental Illness.") If not successfully addressed when they initially present themselves, early risk factors and associated negative behaviors can lead to greater risks later in childhood and in adolescence, such as academic failure and social and emotional difficulties, all of which put an individual at increased risk for substance abuse.

Substance Abuse and Mental Illness

The relationship between substance abuse and other psychiatric disorders can be complex. Although the causal relationships are not fully understood, it is likely that shared genetic or biological risk factors give rise to both substance use disorders and mental illness and that symptoms of one may influence the development of the other, partly because they may affect the same or related brain circuitry and processes—for example, memory and neuroplasticity (Pittenger, 2013). Thus, just as early manifestations of mental illness increase the risk of later substance use, many childhood risk factors for substance use also may increase risk for later appearance of other psychiatric and behavioral problems, including conduct disorder, depression, and delinquency. And substance use during adolescence may also precipitate or affect the course of mental illness—for instance, adolescent use of marijuana may trigger psychosis in individuals with a genetic vulnerability for schizophrenia (Di Forti et al., 2012).

## What if a child has multiple risk factors?

Research has shown that the more risk factors a child has or is exposed to, the more likely it is that he or she will experience problems (see "Accumulated Risk") Unfortunately, many risk factors are related and tend to cluster together. For example, child maltreatment is associated with other family-level risk factors, such as poor parenting skills and parental substance abuse and mental illness (National Research Council and Institute of Medicine, 2009); ongoing maltreatment also results in developmental delays, which can compound a child's risk for later behavioral and emotional problems.

Another example is poverty, which reduces a family's material resources for providing good food, medical care, and child care and thus is often linked with other risk factors such as premature birth and poor nutrition (Gershoff et al., 2003). Poverty may also be linked to problems with attachment, because it reduces the time and energy parents can devote to interacting with their child. As a result, children from impoverished families may encounter multiple risk factors in a variety of developmental contexts.

*Parents and educators should keep in mind that most individuals, even those with risk factors for drug abuse, do not actually develop substance abuse or other mental, emotional, or behavioral problems.*

However, individuals differ widely in how vulnerable they are to being affected by specific risk factors. Parents and educators should keep in mind that most young people, even those with risk factors for substance abuse, do not actually develop drug problems or other mental, emotional, or behavioral problems. *Resilient* children may even have a large number of risk factors but still not experience difficulties (see "Resilience").

## Accumulated Risk

It is possible that children whose personal characteristics and family and school environments are highly protective can still succumb to the effects of accumulated risk if they live in areas with high levels of risk, such as the accumulated stress associated with living in a violent environment. There is as yet no direct evidence supporting this principle in the age group considered in this guide, but evidence from a study on risk and protective factors among a sample of 6th- through 12th-grade students in a five-state survey pointed to the existence of a threshold over which the ability to tolerate risk diminishes. Youth with highest levels of risk factors exhibited increased prevalence rates of problem behaviors, even when they had high levels of protective factors (Pollard et al., 1999).

## Resilience

A major conclusion from research on risk and protective factors among children is that there are some children who, despite having a significant number of risk factors, do not develop problem behaviors. Intervention developers and researchers use findings from protective factor and resiliency research to inform their decisions about what child, parent, and other resources and skills should be addressed through early childhood prevention interventions (Masten, 2011; Masten 2012).

As with risk factors, certain protective factors are important during particular developmental periods:

- *Prenatal Period:* **Good maternal nutrition** is important for the developing fetus, as it can reduce the chances for nutrient-related birth defects (such as spina bifida) and can increase the likelihood that the child will have **normal birth weight**.
- *Infancy and Toddlerhood:* Parents who are **highly responsive** to their infant set the stage for strong parent-child attachment.
- *Preschool:* Increasing **behavioral control** in the preschool years improves social competence across the transition to elementary school.
- *Transition to School:* **School readiness** supports mastery of basic concepts (colors, numbers, letters, pre-reading) during kindergarten, setting the stage for academic success throughout the school years.

Protective factors, like risk factors, may be either internal to the individual child or may be qualities of their contexts, including family, school, and community. Internal factors that offer protection across all ages include **intelligence** and **easy temperament** (i.e., adapting well to eating and sleeping schedules and to other new experiences, as well as a generally positive mood) (Masten, 2004; Masten, 2001). Children with an easy temperament are able to make positive adaptations to a variety of situations and may thereby relax parents who are stressed. They may be less susceptible to the impact of parents who have other risk factors, such as being highly disorganized, being overly organized and scheduled, or having a negative mood. (The mix of temperaments among family members and how well they "fit" or match onto one another can greatly influence family climate and functioning.)

External factors important in building a context for healthy development across childhood (Masten, 2004; Masten, 2001) include parenting that includes **warmth**, **consistency**, **age-appropriate expectations**, **praise for accomplishments** (e.g., using the toilet), and **consistent routines and rules**. When providing such an environment does not come naturally to parents, prevention interventions can help them to build the knowledge and skills important for healthy development and the prevention of subsequent problem behaviors such as drug abuse.

Throughout childhood, both at home and at school, it is also important that children be provided both **opportunities for social interaction with peers**—as playing with other children promotes healthy socialization—and **opportunities for physical exercise.** Physical activity promotes not only physical health but also cognitive and brain development, including the development of executive control (Hillman et al., 2014; Chaddock-Heyman et al., 2014).

Similar to risk factors, protective factors tend to cluster. For example, sensitive, responsive parenting tends to occur along with other environments that promote good social interactions with peers, school readiness, and behavioral control. Generally, an accumulation of protective factors predicts positive outcomes. But just as having many risk factors does not make substance abuse inevitable, having many protective factors does not ensure an absence of problems.

## Selected References

Aarons GA, Monn AR, Hazen AL, et al. Substance involvement among youths in child welfare: the role of common and unique risk factors. *Am J Orthopsychiatry*. 2008;78(3):340-349.

Ainsworth MS, Blehar MC, Waters E, Wall S. *Patterns of Attachment: A Psychological Study of the Strange Situation.* Hillsdale, NJ: Erlbaum; 1978.

Bowlby J. *Attachment and Loss: Volume 1: Attachment.* London: Hogarth Press and the Institute of Psycho-Analysis; 1969.

Bowlby J. *Attachment and Loss: Volume 1: Attachment.* 2nd ed. New York, NY: Basic Books; 1982.

Brown DW, Anda RF, Tiemeier H, et al. Adverse childhood experiences and the risk of premature mortality. *Am J Prev Med.* 2009;37(5):389-396.

Catalano RF, Haggerty KP, Hawkins JD, Elgin J. Prevention of substance use and substance use disorders: role of risk and protective factors. In: Kaminer Y and Winters KC, eds., *Clinical Manual of Adolescent Substance Abuse Treatment.* Arlington, VA: American Psychiatric Publishing; 2011.

Chaddock-Heyman L, Hillman CH, Cohen NJ, Kramer AF. III. The importance of physical activity and aerobic fitness for cognitive control and memory in children. *Monogr Soc Res Child Dev.* 2014;79(4):25-50.

Cowen E, Work W. Resilient children, psychological wellness, and primary prevention. *Am J Community Psychol.* 1988;16(4):591-607.

Di Forti M, Iyegbe C, Sallis H, et al. Confirmation that the AKT1 (rs2494732) genotype influences the risk of psychosis in cannabis users. *Biol Psychiatry.* 2012;72:811-816.

Enoch MA. The influence of gene-environment interactions on the development of alcoholism and drug dependence. *Curr Psychiatry Rep.* 2012;14:150-158.

Fearon RP, Bakermans-Kranenburg MJ, van Ijzendoorn MH, Lapsley AM, Roisman GI. The significance of insecure attachment and disorganization in the development of children's externalizing behavior: a meta-analytic study. *Child Dev.* 2010;81(4):435-456.

Garmezy N. Stress-resistant children: The search for protective factors. In: Stevenson JE, ed. *Recent Research in Developmental Psychopathology.* Journal of Child Psychology and Psychiatry (Book Suppl.); 1985:213-233.

Gershoff ET, Aber JL, Raver CC. Child poverty in the U.S.: an evidence-based conceptual framework for programs and policies. In: Jacobs F, Lerner RM, Wertleib D, eds. *Handbook of Applied Developmental Science: Promoting Positive Child, Adolescent, and Family Development through Research, Policies, and Programs* (Vol. 2). Thousand Oaks, CA: Sage; 2003:81-136.

Goldsmith HH, Buss AH, Plomin R, et al. Roundtable: what is temperament? Four approaches. Child Dev. 1987;58(2):505-529.

Gregg L, Barrowclough C, Haddock G. Reasons for increased substance use in psychosis. *Clin Psychol Rev.* 2007;27(4):494-510.

Hawkins JD, Catalano RF, Miller JY. Risk and protective factors for alcohol and other drug problems in adolescence and early adulthood: implications for substance abuse prevention. *Psychol Bull.* 1992;112(1):64-105.

Hillman CH, Pontifex MB, Castelli DM. 2014. Effects of the FITKids randomized controlled trial on executive control and brain function. *Pediatrics.* 2014;134(4):e1063-e1071.

Institute of Medicine and National Research Council. *From Neurons to Neighborhoods: An Update: Workshop Summary.* Washington, DC: The National Academies Press; 2012.

Jackson C, Dickinson D. Enabling parents who smoke to prevent their children from initiating smoking: results from a 3-year intervention evaluation. *Arch Pediatr Adolesc Med.* 2006;160(1):56-62.

Kendler KS, Prescott CA, Myers J, et al. The structure of genetic and environmental risk factors for common psychiatric and substance use disorders in men and women. *Arch Gen Psychiatry.* 2003;60:929-937.

Kessler RC, Berglund P, Demler O, Jin R, Merikangas KR, Walters EE. Lifetime prevalence and age-of-onset distributions of DSM-IV disorders in the National Comorbidity Survey Replication. *Arch Gen Psychiatry.* 2005;62(6):593-602.

Kochanska G, Kim S. Difficult temperament moderates links between maternal responsiveness and children's compliance and behavior problems in low-income families. *J Child Psychol Psychiatry.* 2013;54(3):323-332.

Kochanska G, Kim S. Toward a new understanding of legacy of early attachments for future antisocial trajectories: evidence from two longitudinal studies. Dev Psychopathology. 2012;24(3):783-806.

Lee CL, Bates JE. Mother-child interaction at age two years andperceived difficult temperament. *Child Dev.* 1985;56(5):1314-1325.

Leonardi-Bee J, Jere ML, Britton J. Exposure to parental and sibling smoking and the risk of smoking uptake in childhood and adolescence: a systematic review and meta-analysis. *Thorax.* 2011;66(10):847-855.

Maslowsky J, Schulenberg JE, Zucker RA. Influence of conduct problems and depressive symptomatology on adolescent substance use: developmentally proximal versus distal effects. *Dev Psychol.* 2014;50:1179-1189.

Masten AS. Ordinary magic: resilience processes in development. *Am Psychol.* 2001;56(3):227-238.

Masten AS. Regulatory processes, risk, and resilience in adolescent development. *Ann N Y Acad Sci.* 2004;1021:310-319.

Masten AS. Resilience in children threatened by extreme adversity: frameworks for research, practice, and translational synergy. *Dev Psychopathol.* 2011;23(2):493-506.

Masten AS. Resilience in children: vintage Rutter and beyond. In: Slater A, Quinn P, eds. *Developmental Psychology: Revisiting the Classic Studies.* London, UK: Sage; 2012: 204-221.

Masten AS. Resilience in development: implications of the study of successful adaptation for developmental psychopathology. In: Cicchetti D, ed. *The Emergence of a Discipline: Rochester Symposium on Developmental Psychopathology.* Vol. 1. Hillsdale, NJ: Lawrence Erlbaum Associates, Inc.; 1989:261-294.

McEwen B. Stress and the central role of the brain. Paper presented at *From Neurons to Neighborhoods Anniversary: Ten Years Later.* Washington, DC, October 28, 2010.

National Research Council and Institute of Medicine. *Preventing Mental, Emotional, and Behavioral Disorders Among Young People: Progress and Possibilities.* Committee on the Prevention of Mental Disorders and Substance Abuse Among Children, Youth, and Young Adults: Research Advances and Promising Interventions. Mary Ellen O'Connell, Thomas Boat, and Kenneth E. Warner, eds. Board on Children, Youth, and Families, Division of Behavioral and Social Sciences and Education. Washington, DC: The National Academies Press; 2009.

Noll RB, Zucker RA, Greenberg GS. Identification of alcohol by smell among preschoolers: evidence for early socialization about drugs occurring in the home. *Child Dev.* 1990;61(5):1520-1527.

Padrón A, Galán I, García-Esquinas E, Fernández, Ballbè M, Rodríguez-Artalejo F. Exposure to secondhand smoke in the home and mental health in children: a population-based study. *Tob. Control.* 2015.

Pagani LS. Environmental tobacco smoke exposure and brain development: the case of attention deficit/hyperactivity disorder. *Neurosci. Biobehav. Rev.* 2014;44:195-205.

Pittenger C. Disorders of memory and plasticity in psychiatric disease. *Dialogues Clin Neurosci.* 2013;15(4):455-463.

Pollard JA, Hawkins JD, Arthur MW. Risk and protection: are both necessary to understand diverse behavioral outcomes in adolescence? *Soc Work Res.* 1999;23(3):145-158.

Raposa EB, Hammen CL, Brennan PA, O'Callaghan FO, Naiman JM. Early adversity and health outcomes in young adulthood: the role of ongoing stress. *Health Psychol.* 2014;33(5):410-418.

Rutter M. Resilience in the face of adversity. Protective factors and resistance to psychiatric disorder. *Br J Psychiatry.* 1985;147(6):598-611.

Schindler A, Bröning S. A review on attachment and adolescent substance abuse: empirical evidence and implications for prevention and treatment. *Subst Abus.* 2015;36(3):304-313.

Shonkoff JP; Garner AS; Committee on Psychosocial Aspects of Child and Family Health; Committee on Early Childhood, Adoption, and Dependent Care; Section on Developmental and Behavioral Pediatrics. The lifelong effects of early childhood adversity and toxic stress. *Pediatrics.* 2012;129(1):e232–e246.

Turner RJ, Lloyd DA. Cumulative adversity and drug dependence in young adults: racial/ethnic contrasts. *Addiction.* 2003;98(3):305-315.

U.S. Department of Health and Human Services (HHS). *The Health Consequences of Involuntary Exposure to Tobacco Smoke: A Report of the Surgeon General.* Atlanta, GA: U.S. Department of Health and Human Services, Centers for Disease Control and Prevention, Coordinating Center for Health Promotion, National Center for Chronic Disease Prevention and Health Promotion, Office on Smoking and Health, 2006.

Werner EE. High-risk children in young adulthood: a longitudinal study from birth to 32 years. *Am J Orthopsychiatry.* 1989;59(1):72-81.

Young SE, Rhee SH, Stallings MC, et al. Genetic and environmental vulnerabilities underlying adolescent substance use and problem use: general or specific? *Behav Genet.* 2006;36:603-615.

Zhou S, Rosenthal DG, Sherman S, Zelikoff J, Gordon T, Weitzman M. Physical, behavioral, and cognitive effects of prenatal tobacco and postnatal secondhand smoke exposure. *Curr Probl Pediatr Adolesc Health Care.* 2014;44(8):219-241.

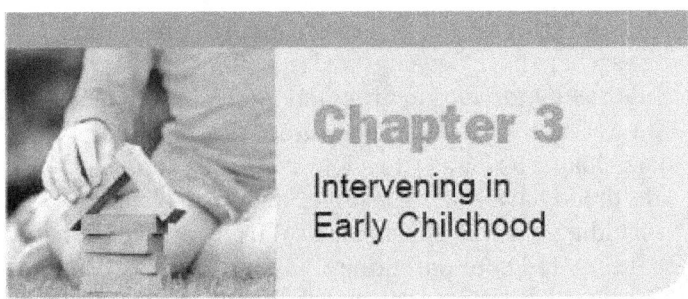

# Chapter 3
## Intervening in Early Childhood

The theoretical rationale for intervening in early childhood is that modifying internal and external risk and protective factors such as those discussed in the previous chapter can influence intermediate or proximal outcomes such as academic and other achievements; effective learning, competence, and skill development; and effective self-regulation. This in turn may reduce the exposure to drugs and the desire to use them during adolescence (see "Logic Model for Intervening in Early Childhood to Prevent Drug Abuse,").

## Logic Model for Intervening in Early Childhood to Prevent Drug Abuse

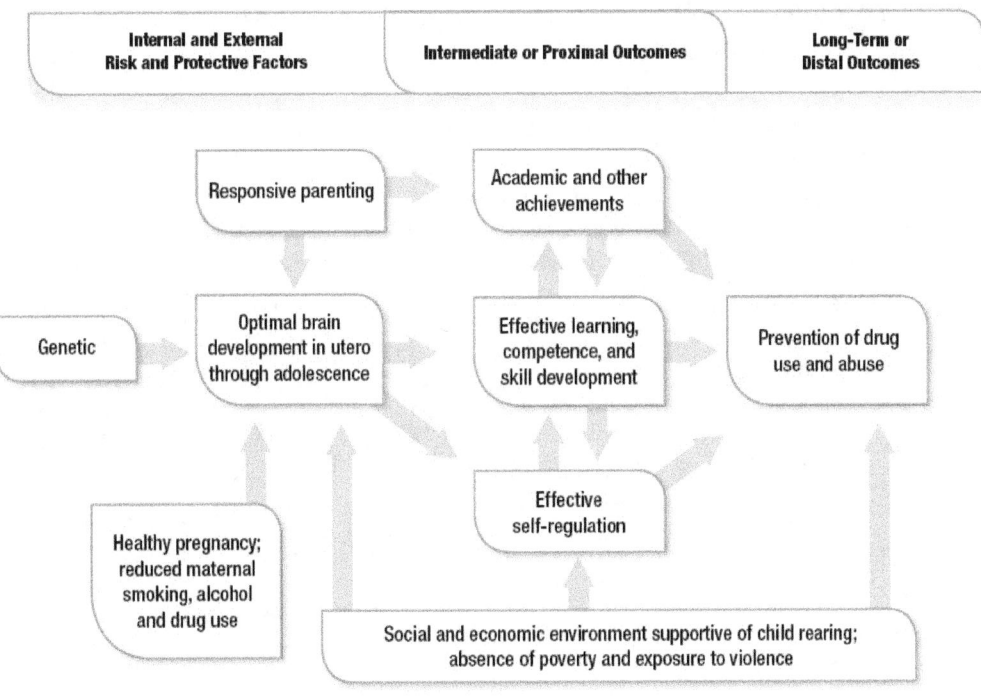

*Principle 3: Intervening early in childhood can have positive long-term effects.*

*Principle 4: Intervening in early childhood can have effects on a wide array of behaviors, even behaviors not specifically targeted by the intervention.*

*Principle 5: Early childhood interventions can positively affect children's biological functioning.*

Following this rationale (or logic model), prevention researchers have developed a large number of early childhood intervention programs, and ample evidence shows that they work. Some studies that followed participants as far as late adolescence or young adulthood have shown positive, long-term effects (including reduced substance use) from interventions that targeted poor parenting skills and other external or internal risk factors during childhood (for an example, see "Intervening to Reduce Risk for Families and Children").

Some of these early interventions have also been found to prevent a wide range of other negative behaviors and promote a wide range of positive behaviors not specifically targeted by the intervention. (See "Intervening Early Can Have Long-Term Effects on a Wide Array of Behaviors.") In some cases, studies have shown that early childhood intervention even affected children's biological functioning, such as their sensitivity to stress.

Intervening to Reduce Risk for Families and Children
Prevention interventions have been shown to alter risk factors for families and children. For example, first-time, low-income mothers who received an intervention including home visits during pregnancy and the first two years of life (the Nurse Family Partnership, described in Research-Based Early Intervention Substance Abuse Programs) had fewer child maltreatment reports involving them or their children 15 years after birth than mothers who did not receive home visits (Eckenrode et al., 2000). In another study, this home visiting intervention significantly reduced role impairment of mothers due to alcohol or substance use (i.e., impaired functioning with family members, with coworkers, and with friends) (Olds et al., 2010). For biological risk, a substance abuse prevention intervention for adolescent African American rural youth and their families (Strong African American Families), designed to strengthen family interactions, was found to be protective for children with genetic risk for initiating high-risk behaviors (Brody et al., 2009).

**Intervening early can have long-term effects on a wide array of behaviors**

| | Intrapersonal | |
|---|---|---|
| **Increased** | Child health | Olds et al., 1986; Olds et al., 1994 |
| | Normalization of cortisol levels | Fisher et al., 2007 |
| | Language development and cognitive function | Olds et al., 2002a; Olds et al., 1994; Lunkenheimer et al., 2008 |
| | Self-regulation (emotional and behavioral control) | Hawkins et al., 2005; Conduct Problem Prevention Research Group, 2002; Lunkenheimer et al., 2008; Reid et al., 1999; Reid et al., 2007 |
| | Pro-social behavior | Catalano et al., 2003; Washburn et al., 2011 |
| | Social competence | Conduct Problem Prevention Research Group, 2002; Webster-Stratton et al., 2008; August et al., 2002; Tolan et al., 2004 |
| | Age at first sexual experience | Lonczak et al., 2002 |
| **Decreased** | Irritability as baby | Olds et al., 1986 |
| | Attention deficit hyperactivity disorder (ADHD) | Tolan et al., 2004 |
| | Internalizing behaviors and disorders (depression, anxiety) | Hawkins et al., 2005; Shaw et al., 2009; Conduct Problem Prevention Research Group, 2002; Izzo et al., 2005; Dolan et al., 1993; Barrera et al., 2002 |
| | Early aggressive behavior | Stoolmiller et al., 2000; Tolan et al., 2004; Tolan et al., 2009; August et al., 2001; August et al., 2003; Dolan et al., 1993; Kellam et al., 1994; Reid et al., 1999 |
| | Externalizing behaviors and disorders (aggression, anti-social behavior, and conduct problems) | Catalano et al., 2003; Reid et al., 2007; Webster-Stratton et al., 2008; Reid et al., 1999; Kellam et al., 2008; Shaw et al., 2009; Kellam et al., 1994; Petras et al., 2008; Barrera et al., 2002; Dishion et al., 2014 |
| | Delinquent, violent, and criminal behaviors | Hawkins et al., 1999; Beets et al., 2009 |
| | Driving under the influence of alcohol | Haggerty et al., 2006 |
| | Likelihood of selling drugs | Hawkins et al., 2005 |
| | Teen pregnancy | Lonczak et al., 2002 |
| | Lifetime sexual partners | Hawkins et al., 1999; Olds et al., 1998; Beets et al., 2009 |
| | Sexually transmitted infection (STI) | Lonczak et al., 2002 |
| | Initiation of tobacco, alcohol and/or other drug use/abuse | Beets et al., 2009; Degarmo et al., 2009; Storr et al., 2002; Wang et al., 2009; Hawkins et al., 1999; Furr-Holden et al., 2004 |
| | Alcohol, tobacco, and other drug use | Brown et al., 2005; Kellam et al., 2008; Furr-Holden et al., 2004; Izzo et al., 2005; Beets et al., 2009; Hawkins et al., 1999 |
| | Substance abuse disorders | Kellam et al., 2008 |
| | Suicidal ideation and attempts | Hawkins et al., 2005; Wilcox et al., 2008 |
| | Any psychiatric diagnosis | Kellam et al., 2008 |

| Family | | |
|---|---|---|
| **Increased** | Maternal prenatal and perinatal care | Olds et al., 1986; Olds et al., 1994 |
| | Maternal concern, support, nurturing, and monitoring for the child | Olds et al., 1986; Lunkenheimer et al., 2008; Reid et al., 1999; Tolan et al., 2004 |
| | Family problem-solving | Degarmo et al., 2009 |
| | Proactive family management | August et al., 2003 |
| | Parent involvement | Reid et al., 1999 |
| | Maternal graduation rates | Olds et al., 1988 |
| | Maternal work history | Olds et al., 1988 |
| **Decreased** | Prenatal smoking | Olds et al., 1986 |
| | Subsequent pregnancies | Olds et al., 1988; Olds et al., 1997 |
| | Child accidents and poisonings | Olds et al., 1986; Olds et al., 1994 |
| | Child abuse and neglect | Olds et al., 1986; Olds et al., 1994; Olds et al., 1997; Eckenrode et al., 2000 |
| | Domestic violence | Olds et al., 2004 |
| | Parental/caregiver stress | August et al., 2003; Fisher & Stoolmiller, 2008 |
| | Maternal depression | Shaw et al., 2009 |
| | Maternal role impairment due to substance use | Olds et al., 1997; Olds et al., 2010 |

| School/Work | | |
|---|---|---|
| **Increased** | Emphasis on social-emotional teaching | Webster-Stratton et al., 2008 |
| | Teacher reported increase in social skills | Reid et al., 1999 |
| | Academic achievement (reading and math) | Snyder et al., 2010; Catalano et al., 2003; Tolan et al., 2004; Tolan et al., 2009; Gunn et al., 2005; August et al., 2001; Dolan et al., 1993; Hawkins et al., 2005 |
| | Cooperative, team learning style | O'Donnell et al., 1995 |
| | School competence, socialization to school context | August et al., 2001; August et al., 2003 |
| | Commitment to school, school bonding | Catalano et al., 2003; Hawkins et al., 1999 |
| | High school completion | Kellam et al., 2008; Hawkins et al., 2005 |
| | College attendance | Hawkins et al., 2005 |
| | Employment | Hawkins et al., 2005 |
| | Time at present job | Hawkins et al., 2005 |
| **Decreased** | Criticism from teachers | Webster-Stratton et al., 2008 |
| | Disruptive behavior | August et al., 2003 |
| | School absenteeism | Snyder et al., 2010 |

| Service Use | | |
|---|---|---|
| **Increased** | Awareness of community services | Olds et al., 1986 |
| **Decreased** | Social service use (Temporary Assistance to Needy Families; Aid to Families with Dependent Children; other) | Olds et al., 1988; Olds et al., 1997; Olds et al., 2010; Poduska et al., 2008 |
| | Special education | Poduska et al., 2008 |
| | Child Protective Services | Eckenrode et al., 2000 |
| | Mental health and drug abuse services | Izzo et al., 2005; Poduska et al., 2008 |
| | Criminal justice involvement | Olds et al., 1998; Eddy et al., 2003; Poduska et al., 2008 |

## What contexts do early childhood interventions target?

Prevention interventions not only support children's development directly but also support the development of skills and resources of those who care for children in their most important primary contexts—or what is sometimes called their *proximal environments.*

*Principle 6: Early childhood prevention interventions should target the proximal environments of the child.*

The proximal environment during very early development is the family, so prevention interventions for the prenatal through infancy and toddlerhood periods often focus on the parents. When providing an environment that supports healthy early development does not come naturally to new parents, prevention interventions can help them to build the necessary knowledge and skills. Family interventions may be delivered in the home, but that is not universally the case; some may be delivered in social service, community health, or educational settings.

The family remains the most important proximal environment for children, but as a child grows and develops, other contexts outside the family become increasingly important as well. The classroom is an important environment during the preschool and elementary school years, and interventions may focus on things like improving school climate, resources, and policies as well as enhancing teachers' skills and parent-teacher communication. Changing classroom environments from those that react to problem behavior to those that encourage pro-social behavior can be achieved through supporting teacher training in constructive classroom management strategies (see "School Interventions").

Some interventions address multiple contexts such as family and school, with emphasis on communication and collaboration between the two environments, thereby making a consistent prevention effort across contexts to affect the target population(s) of the intervention. In fact, this is a primary strategy of interventions for children 3 years of age and older.

> **Principle 7: Positively affecting a child's behavior through early intervention can elicit positive behaviors in other people, improving the overall social environment.**

Even when children are progressing along the normal course of physical, cognitive, social, and emotional development and achieving age-appropriate milestones, improvements in their proximal environments can further their development.

### School Interventions

Programs targeting children making the transition to elementary school focus on building a repertoire of positive competencies including academic, self-regulation, and social skills. For example, tutoring, especially in reading, is one important focus of prevention programs because reading difficulties during the early elementary years is a strong risk factor for school failure and later drug use. Prevention intervention programs also target social skills that affect the children's relationships with peers and adults outside the family. For example, some approaches used in programs that address social skills development include positive behavior teams, group practice, playground and free play monitoring, and rewarding good behaviors. Incorporating skills development into the natural environment of children allows them to practice these skills with peers. Another frequently used strategy for these interventions is training teachers in classroom management strategies. This approach provides teachers with both the skills for managing children's behaviors and activities for teaching children to manage their own behaviors and emotions, thereby helping children develop self-regulation. Also, approaches that draw on mindfulness-based strategies (e.g., meditation, yoga, martial arts) are being developed and tested for their potential to enhance self-regulation.

## Do early childhood interventions target all children or just those at highest risk?

It depends on the type of intervention. *Universal* interventions are delivered to everyone in the population regardless of risk—for example, all children in a preschool or first-grade classroom or all children in a community. *Selective* interventions are delivered to groups of children who are at risk due to some factor they have in common—for example, children entering elementary school with a low level of self-regulation or ability to pay attention, children living in a high poverty or crime area, or children in the foster care system.[‡]

---

[‡] An additional category, *indicated* interventions, has been defined by the Institute of Medicine (Institute of Medicine (1994). *Reducing Risks for Mental Disorders*. Washington, DC: National Academy Press) but is not relevant to early childhood. In the context of substance abuse prevention, indicated interventions are for individuals who already exhibit drug use but do not meet criteria for drug abuse or addiction.

Some interventions target more than one level of risk. For example, within a universal intervention, screening can be provided to determine who has more severe problems and risks, and then additional services can be provided to those most in need based on that screening. Such programs are called *tiered*, because some people progress from one level of intervention to another.[§] (Research-Based Early Intervention Substance Abuse Prevention Programs reviews universal, selective, and tiered programs.)

## What are some characteristic features of early childhood interventions?

Specific characteristics of early childhood intervention programs are generally related to the developmental period of the child, the specific risk to be addressed, and the people with whom the child interacts in his or her proximal environments. Interventions are generally timed to coincide with the transitions between life course periods, because changes occurring within and around the child during these transitions present particular risk factors, as well as opportunities for enhancing protective factors. (See "Risks Addressed Through Specific Age-Appropriate Strategies.")

### Risks Addressed Through Specific Age-Appropriate Strategies

| | Risk | Intervention Strategy |
|---|---|---|
| **Prenatal** | Maternal substance use before and during pregnancy | Counseling through primary care and referral to treatment |
| | Inadequate prenatal care | In-home nurse visits |
| **Infancy and Toddlerhood** | Inappropriate expectations for children | Parenting class on child development |
| | Harsh discipline | Parenting class on managing child behavior |
| | Insecure attachment | Parent class on developing a warm, supportive relationship |
| **Preschool** | Aggressive behavior | Parent and teacher classes on setting limits and boundaries |
| | Poor emotional control | Preschools that teach social-emotional learning |
| | Delayed school readiness | Preschool programs that highlight basic math and language concepts |
| **Elementary School** | Behavioral problems in the classroom | Training teachers on classroom management |
| | Academic problems | Academic tutoring |
| | Child acting out at school | Developing collaborative relationships between school and home |
| | Poor social skills | Peer social groups |

---

[§] Universal interventions do not group high-risk participants, avoiding an environment in which those at elevated risk are set apart or stigmatized by their status. Moreover, many selective and tiered interventions more directly address the problems that a population is likely to encounter, however these interventions carefully consider such issues as stigma and the risks (e.g., modeling of negative behaviors) and benefits of grouping individuals from a subpopulation.

## Prenatal Period, Infancy, and Toddlerhood

Prevention interventions for the prenatal period and infancy usually focus on very young mothers and families who are at risk due to poverty. The goal is to foster a healthy pregnancy, healthy development of mothers and their children, and a healthy parent-child relationship. Specific programs differ, but they commonly screen mothers for drug use, instruct them in good health care practices, and teach them how to connect to appropriate community services. Programs typically focus on mother-child bonding, using consistent discipline, setting an example of pro-social behavior, and getting the child ready for preschool. Involvement of the father is often encouraged as well.

Some programs access mothers at home during the prenatal period. For example, in order to support mothers, nurse visitors may provide extensive one-on-one instruction during visits (Olds, 2002b). Other programs access mothers and their children through services for low-income families. This strategy supports finding mothers and children in need, assessing their needs, and referring them to available services and programs that meet those specific needs (Shaw et al., 2006).

## Preschool

Similar to programs for younger age groups, programs during the preschool period address the well-being of both caregivers and children and the quality of their relationship, primarily through teaching pro-social parenting practices. Early disruptive behaviors of children are addressed in order to prevent escalation of these behaviors, promote better parent-child bonding (Webster-Stratton et al., 2008), and help the child learn positive ways of relating to others. Preschool programs can incorporate much of the same content as programs for younger age groups (for example, encouragement of pro-social child behavior and consistent contingent-responsiveness and non-abusive limit setting) but within very different contexts (such as school) and with children who have a wide variety of risk factors.

*Core elements of a school-based early childhood intervention include training teachers to establish clear rules and rewards for compliance, teach interactively, and promote cooperative learning in small groups.*

Preschool is a point in time when many children are at risk for or entering child protective placements (Child Welfare Information Gateway, 2013), and these children are at increased risk for multiple problems early and later in life. Thus some interventions specifically target foster parents and children. For example, in the Multidimensional Treatment Foster Care Program for Preschoolers (MTFC-P), maltreated foster children receive individualized services in the home, a preschool setting, and a therapeutic child play group; and foster parents are given training to ensure that they are properly equipped to care for children who may come to them with symptoms of severe stress and unusually difficult behavior challenges.

Transition to School

A significant target of programs aimed at the transition to elementary school is creating strong collaborative ties between families and schools. Evidence indicates that such links facilitate children's adjustment to school, academic achievement, pro-social peer friendships, and self-regulation. A notable characteristic of programs targeting this period of development is the use of interactive techniques such as role-playing, guided play sessions, and small-group practice; research has demonstrated that interactive techniques are more successful than lecture and information only (Tobler, 2000).

A number of programs focus on improving communications between parents and teachers and on providing parents with information and strategies for helping their child cope with the structure and behavioral expectations of the classroom and how to facilitate positive peer interactions.

Research shows that parents can help their children develop skills, competencies, and knowledge specific to the school transition and thereby promote a child's school success.

The elementary school is also a focus of interventions to develop children's school competencies. At the heart of these programs are activities that build a repertoire of positive academic, self-regulation, and social skills. Programs may include tutoring—especially in reading, as reading difficulties in early elementary school is a risk factor for ongoing academic problems and later school failure and drug use. Even if they target similar outcomes, programs may use different strategies: For example, social skills development can be approached through positive behavior teams (seating children with social or behavioral problems with more competent children) (Ialongo et al., 1999), group practice, playground and free-play monitoring, or rewarding of good behaviors.

Teachers are also a focus of interventions for this developmental stage. In such programs, teachers are frequently trained in classroom management strategies. Core elements of a school-based early childhood intervention include training teachers to establish clear rules and rewards for compliance, teach interactively, and promote cooperative learning in small groups. Such an approach is designed to provide teachers with both the skills for managing child behavior and activities for teaching children to manage their own emotions and behaviors, thereby helping children develop self-regulation.

In programs that target multiple actors (such as parents and teachers, or parents and children), the program activities for one actor often reinforce those of another. For example, parents who are taught to respond with consistency and a matter-of-fact, warm tone when their child breaks a rule are likely to elicit a positive change in child behavior. Thus, a program to reduce aggressive behavior in children entering school could include activities and training in classroom management for teachers and instruction in supportive, consistent, contingent-responsive parenting strategies for parents and other caregivers, as well as child-oriented program components aimed at increasing the child's attention and self-regulation within the classroom environment.

Behavioral changes in children and the adults who interact with them can be mutually reinforcing. By positively influencing the child's family or school environment, child behavior can, over time, become more pro-social; this, in turn, can elicit more positive interactions with caregivers and peers, and thereby improve the social environment.

## Who benefits the most from early childhood interventions?

While most children and families benefit from interventions, children at increased risk for later substance abuse due to factors such as early aggressive behavior, poor emotional control, or extreme poverty, generally benefit the most from early childhood interventions.

In addition to children, there is evidence that mothers benefit from the parenting interventions. For example, several studies have shown positive effects on maternal depression, substance use, education, and career attainment.

### Selected References

August GJ, Hektner JM, Egan EA, Realmuto GM, Bloomquist ML. The Early Risers longitudinal prevention trial: examination of 3-year outcomes in aggressive children with intent-to-treat and as-intended analyses. *Psychol Addict Behav.* 2002;14(4, Suppl):S27-S39.

August GJ, Lee SS, Bloomquist L, Realmuto GM, Hektner JM. Dissemination of an evidence-based prevention innovation for aggressive children living in culturally diverse, urban neighborhoods: the Early Risers effectiveness study. *Prev Sci.* 2003;4(4):271-286.

August GJ, Realmuto GM, Hektner JM, Bloomquist ML. An integrated components preventive intervention for aggressive elementary school children: the Early Risers Program. *J Consult Clin Psychol.* 2001;69(4):614-626.

Barrera M, Jr, Biglan A, Taylor TK, et al. Early elementary school intervention to reduce conduct problems: a randomized trial with Hispanic and non-Hispanic children. *Prev Sci.* 2002;3(2):83-94.

Brody GH, Chen YF, Beach SR, Philibert RA, Kogan SM. Participation in a family-centered prevention program decreases genetic risk for adolescents' risky behaviors. *Pediatrics.* 2009;124(3):911-917.

Brown EC, Catalano RF, Fleming CB, Haggerty KP, Abbott RD. Adolescent substance use outcomes in the Raising Healthy Children project: a two-part latent growth curve analysis. *J Consult Clin Psychol.* 2005;73(4):699-710.

Catalano RF, Mazza JJ, Harachi TW, Abbott RD, Haggrety KP, Fleming CB. Raising healthy children through enhancing social development in elementary school: results after 1.5 years. *J Sch Psychol.* 2003;41(2):143-164.

Child Welfare Information Gateway. *Foster Care Statistics, 2011.* Washington, DC: Child Welfare Information Gateway, 2013.

Conduct Problems Prevention Research Group. Evaluation of the first 3 years of the Fast Track Prevention Trial with children at high risk for adolescent conduct problems. *J Abnorm Child Psychol.* 2002;30(1):19-35.

DeGarmo DS, Eddy JM, Reid JB, Fetrow RA. Evaluating mediators of the impact of the Linking the Interests of Families and Teachers (LIFT) multimodal preventive intervention on substance use initiation and growth across adolescence. *Prev Sci.* 2009;10(3):208-220.

Dishion TJ, Brennan LM, Shaw DS, McEachern AD, Wilson MN, Jo B. Prevention of problem behavior through annual family check-ups in early childhood: intervention effects form home to early elementary school. *J Abnorm Child Psychol.* 2014;42(3):343-354.

Dolan LJ, Kellam SG, Brown CH, et al. The short-term impact of two classroom-based preventive intervention trials on aggressive and shy behaviors and poor achievement. *J Appl Dev Psychol.* 1993;14:317-345.

Eckenrode J, Ganzel B, Henderson CR, Jr, et al. Preventing child abuse and neglect with a program of nurse home visitation: the limiting effects of domestic violence. *JAMA.* 2000;284(11):1385-1391.

Eddy JM, Reid JB, Stoolmiller M, Fetrow RA. Outcomes during middle school for an elementary school-based preventive intervention for conduct problems: follow-up results from a randomized trial. *Behav Ther.* 2003;34(4):535-552.

Fisher PA, Stoolmiller M, Gunnar MR, Burraston BO. Effects of a therapeutic intervention for foster preschoolers on diurnal cortisol activity. *Psychoneuroendocrinology.* 2007;32(8–10):892-905.

Fisher PA, Stoolmiller M. Intervention effects on foster parent stress: associations with child cortisol levels. *Dev Psychopathol.* 2008;20(3):1003-1021.

Furr-Holden CDM, Ialongo NS, Anthony JC, Petras H, Kellam SG. Developmentally inspired drug prevention: middle school outcomes in a school-based randomized prevention trial. *Drug Alcohol Depend.* 2004;73(2):149-158.

Gunn B, Smolkowski K, Biglan A, Black C, Blair J. Fostering the development of reading skill through supplemental instruction: results for Hispanic and non-Hispanic students. *J Spec Educ.* 2005;39(2):66-85.

Haggerty KP, Fleming CB, Catalano RF, Harachi TW, Abbott RD. Raising healthy children: examining the impact of promoting healthy driving behavior within a social development intervention. *Prev Sci.* 2006;7(3):257-267.

Hawkins JD, Catalano RF, Kosterman R, Abbott RD, Hill KG. Preventing adolescent health-risk behaviors by strengthening protection during childhood. *Arch Pediatr Adolesc Med.* 1999;153(3):226-234.

Hawkins JD, Kosterman R, Catalano RF, Hill KG, Abbott RD. Promoting positive adult functioning through social development intervention in childhood: long-term effects from the Seattle Social Development Project. *Arch Pediatr Adolesc Med.* 2005;159(1):25-31.

Ialongo NS, Werthamer L, Kellam SG, Brown CH, Wang S, Lin Y. Proximal impact of two first-grade preventive interventions on the early risk behaviors for later substance abuse, depression, and antisocial behavior. *Am J Community Psychol.* 1999;27(5):599-641.

Izzo C, Eckenrode J, Smith E, et al. Reducing the impact of uncontrollable stressful life events through a program of nurse home visitation for new parents. *Prev Sci.* 2005;6(4):269-274.

Kellam SG, Brown CH, Poduska JM, et al. Effects of a universal classroom behavior management program in first and second grades on young adult behavioral, psychiatric, and social outcomes. *Drug Alcohol Depend.* 2008;95(Suppl 1):S5-S28.

Kellam SG, Rebok GW, Ialongo N, Mayer LS. The course and malleability of aggressive behavior from early first grade into middle school: results of a developmental epidemiologically-based preventive trial. *J Child Psychol Psychiatr.* 1994;35(2):259-281.

Lonczak HS, Abbott RD, Hawkins JD, Kosterman R, Catalano RF. Effects of the Seattle Social Development Project on sexual behavior, pregnancy, birth, and sexually transmitted disease outcomes by age 21 years. *Arch Pediatr Adolesc Med.* 2002;156(5):438-447.

Lunkenheimer ES, Dishion TJ, Shaw DS, et al. Collateral benefits of the Family Check-Up on early childhood school readiness: indirect effects of parents' positive behavior support. *Dev Psychopathol.* 2008;44(6):1737-1752.

O'Donnell J, Hawkins JD, Catalano RF, Abbott RD, Day LE. Preventing school failure, drug use, and delinquency among low-income children: long-term intervention in elementary schools. *Am J Orthopsychiatry.* 1995;65(1):87-100.

Olds DL, Eckenrose J, Henderson CR, Jr., et al. Long-term effects of home visitation on maternal life course and child abuse and neglect. Fifteen-year follow-up of a randomized trial. *JAMA.* 1997;278(8):637-643.

Olds DL, Henderson CR Jr., Tatelbaum R, Chamberlin R. Improving the delivery of prenatal care and outcomes of pregnancy: a randomized trial of nurse home visitation. *Pediatrics.* 1986;77(1):16-28.

Olds DL, Henderson CR Jr., Tatelbaum R, Chamberlin R. Improving the life-course development of socially disadvantaged mothers: a randomized trial of nurse home visitation. *Am J Public Health.* 1988;78(11):1436-1445.

Olds DL, Henderson CR, Jr., Cole R, et al. Long-term effects of nurse home visitation on children's criminal and antisocial behavior: 15-year follow-up of a randomized controlled trial. *JAMA.* 1998;280(14):1238-1244.

Olds DL, Henderson CR, Jr., Kitzman H. Does prenatal and infancy nurse home visitation have enduring effects on qualities of parental caregiving and child health at 25 and 50 months of life? *Pediatrics.* 1994;93(1):89-98.

Olds DL, Kitzman H, Cole R, et al. Enduring effects of prenatal and infancy home visiting by nurses on maternal life course and government spending: follow-up of a randomized trial among children at age 12 years. *Arch Pediatr Adolesc Med.* 2010;164(5):419-424.

Olds DL, Robinson J, O'Brien R, et al. Home visiting by paraprofessionals and by nurses: a randomized controlled trial. *Pediatrics.* 2002;110(3):486-496.

Olds DL, Robinson J, Pettitt L, et al. Effects of home visits by paraprofessionals and by nurses: age 4 follow-up results of a randomized trial. *Pediatrics.* 2004;114:1560-1568.

Olds DL. Prenatal and infancy home visiting by nurses: from randomized trials to community replication. *Prev Sci.* 2002;3(3):153-172.

Petras H, Kellam SG, Brown CH, Muthen BO, Ialongo NS, Poduska JM. Developmental epidemiological courses leading to antisocial personality disorder and violent and criminal behavior: effects by young adulthood of a universal preventive intervention in first- and second-grade classrooms. *Drug Alcohol Depend.* 2008;95(Suppl. 1):S45-S59.

Poduska JM, Kellam SG, Wang W, Brown CH, Ialongo NS, Toyinbo P. Impact of the Good Behavior Game, a universal classroom-based behavior intervention, on young adult service use for problems with emotions, behavior, or drugs or alcohol. *Drug Alcohol Depend.* 2008;95(Suppl. 1):S29-S44.

Reid JB, Eddy JM, Fetrow RA, Stoolmiller M. Description and immediate impacts of a preventive intervention for conduct problems. *Am J Community Psychol.* 1999;27(4):483-517.

Reid MJ, Webster-Stratton C, Hammond M. Enhancing a classroom social competence and problem-solving curriculum by offering parent training to families of moderate- to high-risk elementary school children. *J Clin Child Adolesc Psychol.* 2007;36(4):605-620.

Shaw D, Connell A, Dishion T, Wilson M, Gardner F. Improvements in maternal depression as a mediator of intervention effects on early childhood problem behavior. *Dev Psychopathol.* 2009;21(2):417-439.

Shaw DS, Dishion TJ, Supplee L, Gardner F, Arnds K. Randomized trial of a family-centered approach to the prevention of early conduct problems: 2-year effects of the family check-up in early childhood. *J Consult Clin Psychol.* 2006;74(1):1-9.

Snyder FJ, Vuchinich S, Acock A, et al. Impact of the Positive Action program on school-level indicators of academic achievement, absenteeism, and disciplinary outcomes: a matched-pair, cluster randomized, controlled trial. *J Res Educ Eff.* 2010;3(1):26-55.

Stoolmiller M, Eddy JM, Reid JB. Detecting and describing preventive intervention effects in a universal school-based randomized trial targeting delinquent and violent behavior. *J Consult Clin Psychol.* 2000;68(2):296-306.

Storr CL, Ialongo NS, Kellam SG, Anthony JC. A randomized controlled trial of two primary school intervention strategies to prevent early onset tobacco smoking. *Drug Alcohol Depend.* 2002;66(1):51-60.

Tobler NS. Lessons learned. *Journal of Primary Prevention.* 2000;20:261-274.

Tolan P, Gorman-Smith D, Henry D. Supporting families in a high-risk setting: proximal effects of the SAFEChildren preventive intervention. *J Consult Clin Psychol.* 2004;72(5):855-869.

Tolan PH, Gorman-Smith D, Henry D, Schoeny M. The benefits of booster interventions: evidence from a family-focused prevention program. *Prev Sci.* 2009;10(4): 287-297.

Wang Y, Browne DC, Petras H, et al. Depressed mood and the effect of two universal first grade preventive interventions on survival to the first tobacco cigarette smoked among urban youth. *Drug Alcohol Depend.* 2009;100(3):194-203.

Washburn I, Acock A, Vuchinich S, et al. Effects of a social-emotional and character development program on the trajectory of behaviors associated with social-emotional and character development: findings from three randomized trials. *Prev Sci.* 2011;12(3):314-323.

Webster-Stratton C, Reid MJ, Stoolmiller M. Preventing conduct problems and improving school readiness: evaluation of the Incredible Years Teacher and Child Training Programs in high-risk schools. *J Child Psychol Psychiatry.* 2008;49(5):471-488.

Wilcox HC, Kellam SG, Brown CH, et al. The impact of two universal randomized first- and second-grade classroom interventions on young adult suicide ideation and attempts. *Drug Alcohol Depend.* 2008;95(Suppl. 1):S60-S73.

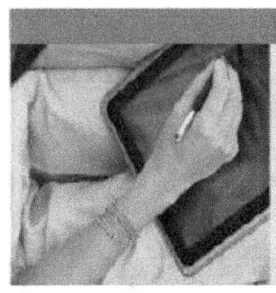

# Chapter 4

## Research-Based Early Intervention Substance Abuse Prevention Programs

NIDA-supported research over the past 3 decades has resulted in the development of a range of early intervention substance abuse prevention programs that span the prenatal period, infancy and toddlerhood (0 to 3 years), preschool (3 to 6), and the transition to elementary school (6 to 8). The programs described in this chapter are arranged by developmental period. Within each age range, programs are presented according to level of prevention—universal, selective, and tiered. (Not all prevention levels exist within each age range.) Contact information is provided for each of the programs listed. Research findings regarding the specific programs can be found following each program description. (See "NIDA-Funded Early Interventions.")

### NIDA-Funded Early Interventions

**Prenatal/Infancy and Toddlerhood**

| Universal Programs | Target Population | Context | Reference |
|---|---|---|---|
| Durham Connects | Mother, Father (when possible), Child | Family | Dodge et al., 2013a |

| Selective Programs | Target Population | Context | Reference |
|---|---|---|---|
| Early Steps, Family Check Up | Mother, Child | Family | Shaw et al., 2006 |
| Family Spirit | Mother, Child | Family | Mullany et al., 2012 |
| Nurse Family Partnership | Mother, Father (if present), Child | Family | Olds, 2002b |

**Preschool**

| Selective Programs | Target Population | Context | Reference |
|---|---|---|---|
| Multidimensional Treatment Foster Care for Preschoolers | Foster family, Child | Family, School | Fisher & Chamberlain, 2000 |

**Transition to Elementary School**

| Universal Programs | Target Population | Context | Reference |
|---|---|---|---|
| **Caring School Community Program** | School, Teacher, Family, Child | School, Family | Battistich et al., 1997 |
| **Classroom-Centered Intervention** | Classroom, Child | School | Kellam & Rebok, 1992 |
| **Linking the Interests of Families and Teachers** | Classroom, Child, Family | School, Family | Reid et al. 1999 |
| **Raising Health Children** | Family, Child, Classroom | School, Family | Catalano et al., 2003 |
| **SAFEChildren** | Family, Child | School, Family | Tolan et al., 2004 |
| **Seattle Social Development Project** | School, Parent/Family, Child | School, Family | Hawkins et al., 1999 |

| Selective Programs | Target Population | Context | Reference |
|---|---|---|---|
| **Early Risers "Skills for Success" Risk Prevention Program** | Parent, Child | School, Family | August et al., 2001 |
| **Kids in Transition to School** | Child | School | Pears et al., 2007 |

| Tiered Programs | Target Population | Context | Reference |
|---|---|---|---|
| **Fast Track Prevention Trial for Conduct Problems** | Family, School, Class, Child | School, Family, Community | Conduct Problems Prevention Research Group, 2000 |
| **Incredible Years** | Family, Child, Classroom | School, Family | Webster-Stratton et al., 2008 |
| **Positive Action** | Family, School, Class, Child | School | Flay et al., 2001 |
| **Schools and Homes in Partnership** | Parent, Child | School, Family | Barrera et al., 2002 |

## Universal Programs

*Durham Connects.* Durham Connects is a brief, universal postnatal nurse home-visiting program designed to assess family needs and connect parents with community resources to improve infant health and well-being. Important aims are to alleviate parent substance use and other problems and to prevent child abuse. Designed for population-level implementation, it engages every family but rapidly triages and concentrates resources on families with assessed higher needs. The highly structured program consists of four to seven scripted intervention contacts, beginning with consent during a birthing hospital visit when a staff member communicates the importance of community support for parenting, one to three nurse home visits when the infant is between 3 and 12 weeks old, one to two nurse contacts with a community service provider, and a telephone or home follow-up 1 month later.

> **Findings:** In a population-level randomized controlled trial with almost 5,000 families, families assigned to Durham Connects had 50 percent less emergency medical care use across the first 12 months of life than the control group. This population-level program yields similar benefits to other, more intensive nurse visiting programs that have found reductions in service usage in infancy (Dodge et al., 2013b).

**Contact for materials and research:**
Kenneth A. Dodge, Ph.D.
Duke University
Center for Child and Family Policy
Box 90545
Durham, NC 27708-0545
Phone: 919-613-9303
Fax: 919-684-3731
E-mail: dodge@duke.edu
www.childandfamilypolicy.duke.edu

## Selective Programs

*Early Steps, Family Check-Up (Early Steps FCU).* Early Steps FCU is a brief selective intervention designed to support families with young children (ages 2 through 5) who may experience stress due to income or other family circumstances. It is a brief (three-session) family intervention that consists of an initial parent interview followed by family assessment and a feedback session; there is an option for additional follow-up sessions on parent management support using an empirically validated curriculum (Everyday Parenting). Early Steps FCU aims to improve parenting practices, increase the involvement of caregivers with children, and link parents to support services with the goal of preventing the development of childhood problem behaviors. A benefit of this intervention is that it works with individual families to identify specific needs and strengths, thus tailoring the intervention to each family's needs.

> **Findings:** To test the Early Steps FCU, participants were identified through a national family nutrition and health program for young families referred to as the Women, Infants, and Children Nutrition Program (WIC). Early Steps FCU resulted in reduced problem behaviors, especially among the highest risk children. This effect on child behavior was accounted for by improvements in positive parenting. The Early Steps FCU was also found to be associated with attenuated internalizing behavior, increased self-regulation, and improved language skills among children and reduced depressive symptoms in mothers. This highlights that prevention interventions can improve parenting practices and reduce problem behaviors in children, and improve parental functioning (Dishion et al., 2008).

**Contact for materials, research, and support for training:**

Thomas Dishion, Ph.D.
Professor
Department of Psychology
Director
Prevention Research Center
Arizona State University
900 South McAllister Avenue
Tempe, AZ 85287
E-mail: dishion@asu.edu
Phone: 480-965-5405
Fax: 480-965-5430

*Family Spirit.* Family Spirit is a pregnancy and early childhood selective prevention intervention for American Indian teen mothers and their children, delivered by Native paraprofessionals (local workers trained and supervised by professionals to deliver the program) in home visits. Sessions target parenting skills across early childhood (0 to 3 years), maternal substance abuse prevention and life skills, and positive child psychosocial development. The program consists of 43 highly structured lessons, occurring weekly through pregnancy, biweekly in the first 3 months after childbirth, monthly between 4 and 12 months, and bimonthly between 12 and 36 months.

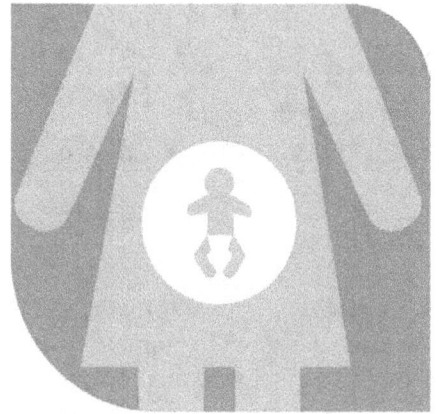

**Findings:** Recent findings for the Family Spirit intervention showed that, at 12 months postpartum, intervention mothers had greater parenting knowledge, parenting self-efficacy, and home safety attitudes with fewer externalizing behaviors (opposition/defiance, rule breaking, and social problems) than the control group. Their children also had fewer externalizing problems. In a sub-sample of mothers with any lifetime substance use at baseline, children of substance users in the intervention versus control group were found to have fewer externalizing and dysregulation problems, and fewer scored in the clinically "at risk" range for externalizing and internalizing problems (Barlow et al., 2006; Barlow et al., 2012).

**Contact for materials and research:**
Allison Barlow, Ph.D.
Johns Hopkins Center for American Indian Health
621 North Washington Street
Baltimore, MD 21205
E-mail: abarlow@jhsph.edu
Phone: 410-614-2072 or 410-294-1362
Fax: 410-955-2010
www.jhsph.edu/caih

*Nurse Family Partnership.* Nurse Family Partnership is a selective prenatal and infancy home visitation program for young first-time mothers from low socio-economic backgrounds and their children through age 2. The program's primary goals are to improve the outcomes of pregnancy by helping pregnant women improve their health, for instance through diet and discontinuing cigarette, alcohol, or other drug use; to improve children's subsequent health and development by promoting competent parental caregiving; and to improve parents' economic self-sufficiency by helping them develop a vision for the future of their families and to make appropriate decisions about completing their educations, finding work, and planning the timing of subsequent pregnancies. The program consists of 64 structured visits beginning as early in pregnancy as possible and continuing through the first 2 years of the child's life. Nurses adapt the content and frequency of visits to meet families' needs and aspirations.

**Findings:** Findings on this program have confirmed that the Nurse Family Partnership (NFP) intervention produces a broad array of positive effects on immediate and intermediate outcomes, including improved maternal, infant, and child health and reduced injuries, neglect, and maltreatment of children. There are also long-term effects on child outcomes. For example, children in the NFP intervention group had lower rates of substance use, delinquency, and involvement in the juvenile justice system at age 12 than control group children. This intervention is effective with diverse populations (e.g., rural and urban) but not as effective when implemented by trained paraprofessionals; hence, nurse participation is a key aspect of this intervention (Kitzman et al., 2010; Olds et al., 2010).

**Contact for information on implementation:**
Nurse-Family Partnership National Service Office
1900 Grant Street
Suite 400
Denver, CO 80203
E-mail: info@nursefamilypartnership.org
Phone: 866-864-5226
Fax: 303-327-4260
www.nursefamilypartnership.org

**Contact for materials and research:**
David L. Olds, Ph.D.
Prevention Research Center for Family and Child Health
University of Colorado Health Sciences Center
1825 Marion Street
Denver, CO 80220
E-mail: david.olds@ucdenver.edu
Phone: 303-724-2892

## Preschool (Ages 3 to 6 Years)

**Selective Programs**

*Multidimensional Treatment Foster Care for Preschoolers (MTFC-P)* (Formerly Early Intervention Foster Care [EIFC]). MTFC-P is a selective intervention for 3- to 6-year-old children in foster care. It attempts to create optimal foster care conditions (including providing responsive and consistent caregiving and predictable daily routines) to facilitate developmental progress and address difficulties related to delayed maturation and behavioral and emotional problems. Children are referred from the child welfare system by their caseworkers. The intervention is delivered by family therapists and licensed psychologists who provide parenting training and access to resources for foster parents above and beyond those offered in regular foster care. Prior to bringing a new foster child into their home, foster parents receive 12 hours of training during which they learn how to concretely encourage pro-social behavior, consistently and non-abusively set limits to address disruptive behavior, and give children close supervision. Foster parents attend weekly support group meetings and have frequent telephone contact with intervention staff, including access to a 24-hour crisis hotline. The children receive weekly individualized skills training services from a child therapist and attend a weekly therapeutic playgroup. In addition, family therapists work with families to facilitate the transition out of foster care and into a permanent home.

**Findings:** Children in this early intervention foster care program showed more secure behaviors, improved response to feedback, and improved sleep. They also showed reduced stress, measured by the level of the hormone cortisol. Over the course of MTFC-P placement, children's cortisol levels normalized and became similar to those of a control group of non-maltreated children living with their biological parents. Another measure of child function among children in foster care is disrupted placement, with children who function better staying in a placement rather than being moved to another foster home. Successful transitions into permanent homes were significantly higher for children in the early intervention foster care program compared to children in regular foster care (Fisher et al., 2007; Fisher et al., 2009).

**Contact for materials and research***:*
Philip A. Fisher, Ph.D.
Oregon Social Learning Center
10 Shelton McMurphey Boulevard
Eugene, OR 97401
E-mail: philf@oslc.org
Phone: 541-485-2711
Fax: 541-485-7087
www.oslc.org, www.oslccp.org

Transition to School (Ages 6 to 8 Years)

## Universal Programs

*Caring School Community Program* (Formerly Child Development Project). This is a universal family and school intervention to reduce risk factors and bolster protective factors among children making the transition to elementary school. The program focuses on strengthening students' "sense of community," or connection to school, which research has shown to be pivotal in reducing drug use, violence, and mental health problems and promoting academic motivation and achievement. The program consists of a set of classroom, school, and family involvement approaches that reinforce the development of skills by children across contexts. These promote positive peer, teacher-student, and home-school relationships and the development of social, emotional, and character-related skills. The program provides detailed instructional, implementation, and staff development materials.

**Findings:** Research results showed a significant reduction in students' drug use and involvement in other problem behaviors in schools where the Caring School Community Program was widely implemented by teachers over a period of 3 years, compared to schools not implementing the program (Battistich et al., 2000).

**Contact for Materials and Research:**
Peter Brunn
Caring School Community Program
Developmental Studies Center
2000 Embarcadero
Suite 305
Oakland, CA 94606
E-mail: Peter_Brunn@devstu.org
Phone: 510-533-0213
Fax: 510-464-3670
www.devstu.org

*Classroom-Centered (CC) Intervention.* The CC Intervention is a multi-component, universal first-grade preventive intervention targeting early aggressive or disruptive behavior and poor academic achievement, with the long-term goal of reducing adolescent and adult antisocial behavior and substance abuse. The CC Intervention enhances teachers' behavior management and instructional skills through the use of an effective classroom behavior management program called the "Good Behavior Game" and an enhanced reading and mathematics curricula.

**Findings:** Results from an ongoing follow-up study indicate that the CC Intervention decreased the level of conduct problems in middle and high school, delayed the onset of smoking tobacco in both males and females, and was associated with an increased likelihood of high school graduation and a lower likelihood of special education use. While broad benefits of this intervention have been found, the effects of the CC Intervention are strongest for males who exhibit a relatively high level of aggressive-disruptive behavior in the early elementary school years, indicating that this universal intervention can have a targeted impact on a high-risk group of children. In a study of the Good Behavior Game, males in the intervention group who were more aggressive in 1st grade had higher rates of high school graduation, lower rates of alcohol and drug abuse and dependence, and lower rates of antisocial personality disorder at ages 19 to 21 than males in the control condition (Bradshaw et al., 2009; Wang et al., 2012).

**Contact for materials and research:**
Nicholas Ialongo, Ph.D.
Department of Mental Health
Johns Hopkins Bloomberg School of Public Health
Johns Hopkins University
624 North Broadway
Baltimore, MD 21205
E-mail: nialongo@jhsph.edu
Phone: 410-955-0414
Fax: 410-955-9088
www.jhsph.edu/prevention

*Linking the Interests of Families and Teachers (LIFT).* LIFT is a universal preventive intervention that was developed for elementary schools in communities with high levels of juvenile delinquency. Created for students in the 1st and 5th grades, LIFT is a multi-component intervention that is designed to improve school and family environments while also reinforcing stronger links between the two. Two school components are designed to decrease the likelihood of both aggressive child behavior and rejection of aggressive children by their peers: A classroom component improves upon social and problem solving skills during 20 1-hour-long sessions, and a playground component based on the Good Behavior Game (see the CC Intervention) reinforces positive social behaviors during free (unstructured) play. There is also a parent management training component emphasizing good discipline, supervision, and problem-solving during a group meeting, once a week for 6 weeks, as well as parent support between sessions. In addition, a school-parent communication component supports connections between the families and teachers through phone, email, and Internet, as well as a weekly newsletter sent to parents describing the LIFT activities of the week and suggesting complementary home activities.

> **Findings:** Within the context of a randomized controlled trial of 12 schools, LIFT resulted in improvements in parenting behaviors and child social skills as well as reduced child physical aggression on the playground. During their middle and high school years, children in schools assigned to the LIFT intervention had lower rates of police arrest and substance use compared to children in control schools (DeGarmo et al., 2009; Eddy et al., 2000).

**Contact for materials and research:**
J. Mark Eddy, Ph.D.
Partners for Our Children
School of Social Work
University of Washington
UW Mailbox 359476
Seattle, WA 98195
E-mail: jmarke@uw.edu
Phone: 206-221-3144
Fax: 206-221-3155
www.partnersforourchildren.org

*Raising Healthy Children (RHC).* RHC is a school- and home-based intervention targeting children in grades 1 through 12. It engages classroom teachers, parents, and students with the goal of increasing pro-social behavior and reducing substance use and other problem behavior by addressing developmentally salient risk and protective factors. Teachers attend workshops to improve instruction and classroom management practices and have access to one-on-one classroom-based coaching to help them implement the techniques they have learned. Parents participate in parenting workshops and brief, individual, in-home sessions as students approach critical transitions in adolescence. Children learn social, emotional, and cognitive skills through classroom, after-school, and parent-youth sessions. In addition, families have access to school-home coordinators (SHCs) who check in with families several times a year and help solve problems that arise.

**Findings:** Students who participated in the RHC intervention showed higher academic performance, a stronger commitment to school, and increased social competency. They also showed lower levels of antisocial behavior and less frequent alcohol and marijuana use, and were less likely to drive under the influence of alcohol or ride with someone who had been drinking alcohol. Reductions in driving under the influence and riding with another driver under the influence were sustained through age 20. As such, the RHC intervention has been shown to promote healthy behaviors and academic achievement, reduce substance use and antisocial behaviors, and reduce drunk driving (Brown et al., 2005; Haggerty et al., 2006).

**Contact for materials and research:**
Kevin Haggerty, Ph.D.
Associate Director, Social Development Research Group
University of Washington School of Social Work
9725 3rd Avenue NE
Suite 401
Seattle, WA 98115
E-mail: haggerty@u.washington.edu
Phone: 206-543-3188
Fax: 206-543-4507
www.sdrg.org

*SAFEChildren.* SAFEChildren is a universal intervention with school and family components developed specifically for 1st graders from urban, disadvantaged, or low-income neighborhoods. This program is designed to help families protect their children from the risks of growing up in communities with high levels of poverty and crime and few social and economic resources. SAFEChildren also specifically focuses on helping inner-city parents manage a child's transition to school with the goal of promoting academic achievement and overall child well-being. The family component brings multiple families together in a group setting once a week for 22 weeks. During these meetings, families receive information about parenting skills, family relationships, and understanding and managing developmental and situational challenges. In addition, there are opportunities to practice skills and solve problems as a group. These multiple-family groups increase support among parents and help families become more engaged with the school and more engaged in managing issues such as problems in the neighborhood. The school component consists of a tutoring program that takes place twice weekly for 22 weeks and emphasizes phonetics as well as a step-by-step advancement in academic skills.

> **Findings:** The SAFEChildren intervention has been shown to improve reading level overall. Among higher-risk families, characterized by poorer family relationships and parenting practices, the SAFEChildren intervention led to improved parental monitoring and reduced child aggression. Furthermore, higher-risk children, characterized by greater aggression and hyperactivity as well as poorer concentration, showed greater reduction in aggression and hyperactivity as well as improved leadership skills. Also, SAFEChildren had an effect on ADHD symptoms from first grade to fourth grade, with intervention children less likely to be rated as high on impulsivity and hyperactivity, over this time frame (Fowler et al., 2014). An additional version of SAFEChildren was developed for 4th grade to deliver booster sessions. Those assigned to the booster showed lower rates of aggression than those with only 1st-grade intervention (Tolan et al., 2009).

**Contact for materials and research:**
Patrick Tolan, Ph.D.
Youth-Nex: The UVA Center to Promote Effective Youth Development
University of Virginia
400 Emmet Street South
PO Box 400281
Charlottesville, VA 22904
E-mail: pht6t@virginia.edu
Phone: 434-243-9551
Fax: 434-982-6035
www.curry.virginia.edu/youth-nex

*Seattle Social Development Project (SSDP).* SSDP is a universal intervention for elementary school children with a school component and voluntary family component, developed to increase pro-social bonds, strengthen attachments to school, and decrease delinquency. The family component consists of parenting classes that cover family management (1st and 2nd grade), engagement in a child's education (2nd and 3rd grade), and the drug abuse prevention program Preparing for the Drug Free Years (PDFY) (5th and 6th grade). In the school component, teachers are trained to establish clear rules and reward compliance, teach interactively, and promote cooperative learning in small groups. The goal is to increase the students' academic performance as well as social skills and increase contact with pro-social peers. In addition, children are taught interpersonal problem-solving skills to improve communication, decision-making, negotiation, and conflict resolution. SSDP is the original intervention that serves as the basis for the Raising Healthy Children (RHC) intervention.

> **Findings:** The SSDP intervention was associated with reduced aggressive behavior in males and reduced self-destructive behavior in females. It has also been shown to reduce delinquency and alcohol use for both males and females. Females were also less likely to have smoked cigarettes and somewhat less likely to have tried marijuana. Further, there is evidence that SSDP increases attachment to school, cooperative learning, and academic achievement. Intervention effects were strongest among children from lower income households. Long-term effects of the SSDP intervention found that those children who received the intervention had less risky sexual behavior (fewer partners, sexually transmitted infections, and pregnancies, and more condom use), were more likely to graduate high school, were more likely to become gainfully employed, and have less involvement with the criminal justice system (Hawkins et al., 2008).

**Contact for materials and research:**
Karl G. Hill, Ph.D.
Social Development Research Group
School of Social Work
University of Washington
9725 3rd Avenue NE
Suite 401
Seattle, WA 98115
E-mail: khill@uw.edu
Phone: 206-685-3859
Fax: 206-543-4507
www.ssdp-tip.org/SSDP/index.html

## Selective Programs

*Early Risers "Skills for Success" Risk Prevention Program.* Early Risers is an intervention for children at higher risk for the development of serious conduct problems, including the use and misuse of drugs. Elementary school-aged children ages 6 to 10 are selected for the program based on the presence of risk factors including exposure to stressful life experiences and/or early aggressive and disruptive behavior. The program is designed to deflect children from the "early starter" developmental pathway toward normal development by improving their academic competence and behavioral self-regulation and encouraging positive peer affiliations. The program also teaches parenting practices that include discipline, nurturance, and involvement. The Early Risers intervention model includes two child-focused components and two parent- or family-focused components delivered over a 2- to 3-year period. The program includes standard skills curricula as well as strategies tailored to address the individual needs and goals of children and their parents.

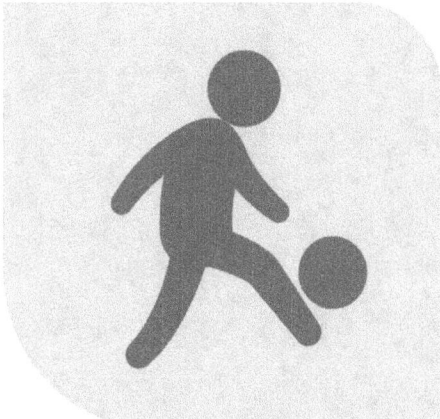

**Findings:** In efficacy and effectiveness trials of Early Risers, program participants have demonstrated greater gains in social skills, peer reputation, pro-social friendship selection, academic achievement, and parent discipline than did controls. The program has been replicated with African-American children. Findings from a 6-year follow-up indicated that the gains in social skills and parent discipline observed early on accounted, in part, for fewer oppositional defiant disorder symptoms among program participants compared with controls in middle school. Recently, in a going-to-scale trial, Early Risers was implemented with high fidelity across 28 school sites, and children made positive gains on outcomes similar to those found in the efficacy trial (August et al., 2003).

**Contact for materials and research:**
Gerald J. August, Ph.D.
Division of Child and Adolescent Psychiatry
University of Minnesota Medical School
P256/2B West
2450 Riverside Avenue
Minneapolis, MN 55454
E-mail: augus001@tc.umn.edu
Phone: 612-273-9711
Fax: 612-273-9779

*Kids in Transition to School (KITS).* KITS is a selective prevention intervention designed to enhance psychosocial and academic readiness in children in the foster care system as they enter school by promoting pre-literacy skills and increasing their attention, effortful control, and social skills in classroom settings. The program gives caregivers skills for facilitating their children's successful transition to kindergarten and becoming involved in their children's schooling. The KITS intervention targets specific school-related skills during the summer before and the first weeks of kindergarten via a therapeutic playgroup; caregiver psycho-educational support groups; and behavioral consultation in the home, school, and community settings.

> **Findings:** Recent findings from a randomized controlled trial of KITS showed positive effects on outcomes in childhood that are linked to later risk for drug use. Children who received the KITS intervention had lower levels of oppositional and aggressive behaviors in the classroom. Also, there were positive intervention effects on early literacy and self-regulatory skills (Pears et al., 2013; Pears et al., 2012).

**Contact for materials and research:**
Katherine Pears, Ph.D.
Oregon Social Learning Center
10 Shelton McMurphey Boulevard
Eugene, OR 97401
E-mail: katherinep@oslc.org
Phone: 541-485-2711
Fax: 541-485-7087
www.oslc.org

## Tiered Programs

*Fast Track Prevention Trial for Conduct Problems.* Fast Track is a tiered comprehensive preventive intervention delivered in grades 1 through 10 to children at high risk for long-term antisocial behavior. Based on a developmental model, the intervention includes a universal classroom program (adapted from the Promoting Alternative Thinking Strategies [PATHS] curriculum) delivered in elementary school. This classroom intervention builds skills in emotional understanding and communication, friendship, self-control, and social problem-solving. In addition, the program includes selective interventions for high-risk children displaying elevated aggression at home and school, as assessed in kindergarten. These high-risk children receive social skills training and academic tutoring, and their parents receive group parent training and individual home visits. Child-focused skill training targets academic and social competencies as well as self-control skills. Parent training builds parents' self-control and targets skills to support the child's school adjustment, improve the child's behavior, promote appropriate expectations for the child's behavior, and improve parent-child interaction.

**Findings:** By the end of 12th grade, the Fast Track intervention was found to reduce adolescent delinquency as indicated by youth self-reports and official arrest records and, for the youths at highest risk, to reduce lifetime prevalence for conduct disorder, oppositional defiant disorder, attention deficit hyperactivity disorder, and any externalizing disorder. At the end of elementary school, children in Fast Track were found to have significantly reduced home and community problems, which included past-year involvement in substance use behaviors. There was no significant effect of the intervention on the onset of delinquent acts that included selling controlled substances. By the end of 12th grade, children in Fast Track had significantly fewer visits to general health providers, pediatric providers, and emergency departments for emotional, behavioral, academic, drug, or alcohol problems. At age 25 years, assignment to intervention significantly decreased the probability of alcohol abuse, marginally decreased binge drinking, did not affect heavy marijuana use, and significantly decreased serious substance use (Conduct Problems Prevention Research Group, 2011; Conduct Problems Prevention Research Group, 2015).

**Contact for materials and research for Fast Track:**
Fast Track & Fast Track Data Center
Bay C, 2nd Floor, Mill Building
2024 West Main Street
Duke Box 90539
Durham, NC 27708
E-mail: www.fasttrackproject.org/contact.php
Phone: 814-865-3879
Fax: 814-865-3246
www.fasttrackproject.org

**Contact for materials for PATHS:**
Channing Bete Company
One Community Place
South Deerfield, MA 01373
E-mail: PrevSci@channing-bete.com
Phone: 877-896-8532
Fax: 800-499-6464
www.channing-bete.com

**Contact for research for PATHS:**
Mark T. Greenberg, Ph.D.
Prevention Research Center
Pennsylvania State University
110 Henderson Building South
University Park, PA 16802
E-mail: mxg47@psu.edu
Phone: 814-863-0112
Fax: 814-865-2530

www.episcenter.psu.edu/ebp/altthinking

**Contact for training for PATHS:**
Carol A. Kusché, Ph.D.
PATHS Training, LLC
927 10th Avenue East
Seattle, WA 98102
E-mail: ckusche@comcast.net
Phone and Fax: 206-323-6688
www.pathstraining.com

*Incredible Years® Parents, Teachers, and Children's Training Series.* The Incredible Years series is a tiered, multi-component prevention and treatment intervention implemented in day care, preschool (2 to 5 years), and early primary grades (6 to 8 years). The prevention version of the program can be offered in high-risk schools or day care centers to all parents, teachers, and children; or parents and teachers may identify children at moderate or higher risk based on elevated behavior problem ratings. The treatment version is used for children identified as having behavioral or conduct problems. The comprehensive intervention consists of a parent training component as well as school-based teacher training and child training components.

The **Incredible Years parenting program**
instructs parents in child-directed play, academic and persistence coaching, social and emotional coaching, use of praise and tangible incentives, and positive discipline methods that promote positive relationships and strengthen children's language development, social and emotional competence, school readiness skills, problem-solving, and anger management. Different parent curricula are available for different child developmental stages and teach parents how to partner with day care providers and teachers to develop individualized behavior plans. The program consists of weekly, 2-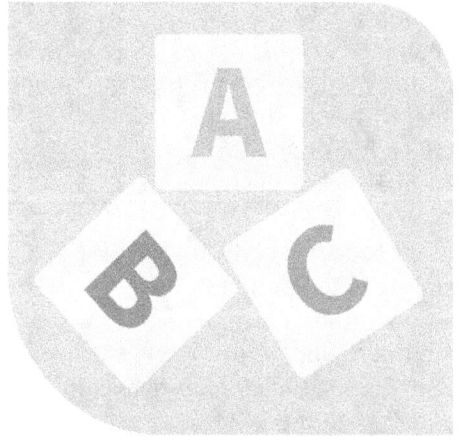
hour parent group meetings with a group leader and/or counselor for a total of 14 to 18 sessions or more. The number of sessions varies according to the child's age, the parent's needs, and whether the prevention or treatment version of the program is being used.

The **Incredible Years child program**, also called the Dina Dinosaur Social Skills Program for young children (Dinosaur School), teaches children school rules, strategies for success in school, feelings literacy, empathy training and emotional regulation, problem-solving skills, and friendship skills. The prevention version of this program can be delivered by classroom teachers throughout the school year two to three times per week, with structured circle time lesson plans and hands-on small group activities. The program uses developmentally appropriate lesson plans for children in preschool through 2nd grade (3 to 8 years old).

The **Incredible Years teacher classroom management program** trains teachers in effective classroom management strategies as well as ways to collaborate with parents to promote consistency of learning from school to home. This program can be delivered to all teachers in a school or to selected teachers who have particularly challenging children in their classrooms. The training is group-based and delivered in six day-long sessions once a month throughout the year, accompanied by individual coaching within the schools.

> **Findings:** Each of the Incredible Years programs has been researched in their prevention and treatment versions. Parent programs consistently result in higher rates of positive parenting behaviors and fewer child behavior problems at home. The child program results in improved social interactions and problem-solving with peers, increased in-school readiness behaviors, and decreased aggression and negative behavior with peers. The teacher program results in increased use of positive classroom management strategies, less negative or critical teaching, more focus on providing children with social emotional curriculum, and increased home-school collaboration (Webster-Stratton & Reid, 2010; Webster-Stratton et al., 2004).

**Contact for materials and research:**
Lisa St. George
Administrator Director
Incredible Years
1411 8th Avenue West
Seattle, WA 98119
E-mail: lisastgeorge@comcast.net
Phone and fax: 206-285-7565
www.incredibleyears.com

*Positive Action (PA).* The PA intervention is a tiered, multi-component, school-based, social-emotional and character development program designed to improve academics and pro-social behaviors as well as decrease problem behaviors. Components of this intervention target the classroom and the overall school climate as well as families and the community. The classroom component consists of grade-specific curricula, which can be implemented beginning as early as Pre-K and extending through grade 12. The lessons cover six broad categories: self-concept, physical and intellectual actions, social/emotional actions for managing oneself responsibly, getting along with others, being honest with oneself and others, and continuous self-improvement. The overall school climate supports the classroom curriculum through ongoing reinforcement of positive behaviors, posters, assemblies, newsletters, and other means. In addition, school counselors work with selected higher-risk students and families to develop PA skills. The family component provides caregivers with resources that parallel the classroom curricula to further reinforce the messages children are receiving at school. The PA intervention also helps establish media messages and civic engagement activities for the larger community in which the children live.

**Findings:** Children who participated in the PA program had improved academic achievement and lower rates of substance use, violence, sexual activity, and absenteeism. Furthermore, the effects of PA on child outcomes increase with multiple years of exposure to the program (Beets et al., 2009; Flay & Allred, 2010; Snyder et al., 2010).

**Contact for materials and research:**
Positive Action, Inc.
264 4th Avenue South
Twin Falls, ID 83301
E-mail: info@positiveaction.net
Phone: 800-345-2974
Fax: 208-733-1590
www.positiveaction.net

*School and Homes in Partnership (SHIP).* The SHIP intervention is a tiered intervention for children in kindergarten through 3rd grade who have aggressive behavior problems or reading difficulties. It is implemented over the course of 2 academic years and includes parent training, a social behavior intervention, and reading instruction. The parent training component is administered in either Spanish or English and consists of the Incredible Years parenting program delivered over 12 to 16 sessions. There are two components to the social behavior intervention. The first component, Contingencies for Learning Academic and Social Skills (CLASS), involves the child working directly with a trained consultant, then the teacher, and lastly the teacher and parents to reduce acting out and improve appropriate classroom behavior. The second component is the Dina Dinosaur Social Skills Program (see Incredible Years), a 2-hour after-school program using puppets and video tapes to model appropriate behavior to children. The reading instruction component consists of daily small-group instruction in phonemic awareness, sound-letter correspondence, and blending. Additional instruction is provided for those students who are still non-readers in the 3rd and 4th grades.

**Findings:** SHIP has been evaluated among both European-American and Hispanic children. It was found to reduce aggressive or anti-social behavior, particularly for those children with early aggressive behavior problems. SHIP has also been found to improve reading abilities (Gunn et al., 2005; Smolkowski et al., 2005).

**Contact for materials and research:**
Anthony Biglan
Oregon Research Institute
1776 Millrace Drive
Eugene, OR 97403
E-mail: tony@ori.org
Phone: 541-484-2123
Fax: 541-484-1108
www.ori.org

## Selected References

August GJ, Lee SS, Bloomquist L, Realmuto GM, Hektner JM. Dissemination of an evidence-based prevention innovation for aggressive children living in culturally diverse, urban neighborhoods: the Early Risers effectiveness study. *Prev Sci.* 2003;4(4):271-286.

August GJ, Realmuto GM, Hektner JM, Bloomquist ML. An integrated components preventive intervention for aggressive elementary school children: the Early Risers Program. *J Consult Clin Psychol.* 2001;69(4):614-626.

Barlow A, Mullany M, Neault N. Effect of a paraprofessional home visiting intervention on American Indian teen mothers' and infants' behavioral risks: a randomized controlled trial. *Am J Psychiatry.* 2012;170(1):83-93.

Barlow A, Varipatis-Baker E, Speakman K, et al. 2006. Home-visiting intervention to improve child care among American Indian adolescent mothers: a randomized trial. *Arch Pediatr Adolesct Med.* 2006;160(11):1101-1107.

Barrera M, Jr, Biglan A, Taylor TK, et al. Early elementary school intervention to reduce conduct problems: a randomized trial with Hispanic and non-Hispanic children. *Prev Sci.* 2002;3(2):83-94.

Battistich V, Schaps E, Watson M, Solomon D, Lewis C. Effects of the Child Development Project on students' drug use and other problem behaviors. *J Prim Prev.* 2000;21(1):75-99.

Battistich V, Solomon D, Watson M, Schaps E. Caring school communities. *Educ Psychol.* 1997;32(3):137-151.

Beets MW, Flay BR, Vuchinich S, et al. Use of a social and character development program to prevent substance use, violent behaviors, and sexual activity among elementary-school students in Hawaii. *Am J Public Health* 2009;99(8):1438-1445.

Bradshaw C, Zmuda J, Kellam S, Ialongo N. Longitudinal impact of two universal preventive interventions in first grade on educational outcomes in high school. *J Educ Psychol.* 101(4):926–937, 2009.

Brown EC, Catalano RF, Fleming CB, Haggerty KP, Abbott RD. Adolescent substance use outcomes in the Raising Healthy Children project: a two-part latent growth curve analysis. *J Consult Clin Psychol.* 2005;73(4):699-710.

Catalano RF, Mazza JJ, Harachi TW, Abbott RD, Haggrety KP, Fleming CB. Raising healthy children through enhancing social development in elementary school: results after 1.5 years. *J Sch Psychol.* 2003;41(2):143-164.

Conduct Problems Prevention Research Group. Impact of early intervention on psychopathology, crime, and well-being at age 25. *Am J Psychiatry.* 2015;172(1):59-70.

Conduct Problems Prevention Research Group. Merging universal and indicated prevention programs: the Fast Track model. *Addict Behav.* 2000;25(6):913-927.

Conduct Problems Prevention Research Group. The effects of the Fast Track preventive intervention on the development of conduct disorder across childhood. *Child Dev.* 2011;82(1):331-345.

DeGarmo DS, Eddy JM, Reid JB, Fetrow RA. Evaluating mediators of the impact of the Linking the Interests of Families and Teachers (LIFT) multimodal preventive intervention on substance use initiation and growth across adolescence. *Prev Sci.* 2009;10(3):208-220.

Dishion TJ, Connell AM, Weaver CM, Shaw DS, Gardner F, Wilson MN. The Family Check-Up with high-risk indigent families: preventing problem behavior by increasing parents' positive behavior support in early childhood. *Child Dev.* 2008;79(5):1395-1414.

Dodge KA, Goodman WB, Murphy R, O'Donnell K, Sato J. Toward population impact from home visiting. *Zero Three.* 2013;33(3):17-23.

Dodge KA, Goodman WB, Murphy RA, O'Donnell K, Sato J. Randomized controlled trial evaluation of universal postnatal nurse home visiting: impacts on child emergency medical care at age 12-months. *Pediatrics.* 2013;132:S140-S146.

Eddy JM, Reid JB, Fetrow RA. An elementary-school based prevention program targeting modifiable antecedents of youth delinquency and violence: linking the Interests of Families and Teachers (LIFT). *J Emot Behav Disord.* 2000;8(3):165-176.

Fisher PA, Chamberlain P. Multidimensional treatment foster care: a program for intensive parent training, family support, and skill building. *J Emot Behav Disord.* 2000;8:155-164.

Fisher PA, Kim HK, Pears KC. Effects of Multidimensional Treatment Foster Care for Preschoolers (MTFC-P) on reducing permanent placement failures among children with placement instability. *Child youth Serv Rev.* 2009;31(5):541-546.

Fisher PA, Stoolmiller M, Gunnar MR, Burraston BO. Effects of a therapeutic intervention for foster preschoolers on diurnal cortisol activity. *Psychoneuroendocrinology.* 2007;32(8–10):892-905.

Flay BR, Allred, CG. The Positive Action Program: improving academics, behavior, and character by teaching comprehensive skills for successful learning and living. In: Lovat T, Toomey R, Clement N, eds., *International Research Handbook on Values Education and Student Wellbeing.* New York, NY: Springer; 2010:471-501.

Flay BR, Allred CG, Ordway N. Effects of the Positive Action program on achievement and discipline: two matched-control comparisons. *Prev Sci.* 2001;2(2):71-89.

Fowler PJ, Henry DB, Schoeny M, Gorman-Smith D, Tolan PH. Effects of the SAFE Children preventive intervention on developmental trajectories of attention-deficit/hyperactivity disorder symptoms. *Dev Psychopathol.* 2014;26(4Pt 1):1161-1179.

Gunn B, Smolkowski K, Biglan A, Black C, Blair J. Fostering the development of reading skill through supplemental instruction: results for Hispanic and non-Hispanic students. *J Spec Educ.* 2005;39(2):66-85.

Haggerty KP, Fleming CB, Catalano RF, Harachi TW, Abbott RD. Raising healthy children: examining the impact of promoting healthy driving behavior within a social development intervention. *Prev Sci.* 2006;7(3):257-267.

Hawkins JD, Catalano RF, Kosterman R, Abbott RD, Hill KG. Preventing adolescent health-risk behaviors by strengthening protection during childhood. *Arch Pediatr Adolesc Med.* 1999;153(3):226-234.

Hawkins JD, Kosterman R, Catalano R, Hill KG, Abbott RD. Effects of social development intervention in childhood 15 years later. *Arch Pediatr Adolesc Med.* 2008;162(12):1133-1141.

Kellam SG, Rebok GW. Building developmental and etiological theory through epidemiologically based preventive intervention trials. In: McCord J, Tremblay RE, eds. *Preventing Antisocial Behavior: Interventions from Birth through Adolescence.* New York, NY: Guilford Press; 1992:162-195.

Kitzman H, Olds D, Cole R, et al. Enduring effects of prenatal and infancy home visiting by nurses on children: follow-up of a randomized trial among children at age 12 years. *Arch Pediatr Adolesc Med.* 2010;164(5):412-418.

Mullany B, Barlow A, Neault N, et al. The Family Spirit Trial for American Indian teen mothers and their children: CBPR rationale, design, methods, and baseline characteristics. *Prev Sci.* 2012;13(5):504-518.

Olds DL, Kitzman H, Cole R, et al. Enduring effects of prenatal and infancy home visiting by nurses on maternal life course and government spending: follow-up of a randomized trial among children at age 12 years. *Arch Pediatr Adolesc Med.* 2010;164(5):419-424.

Olds DL. Prenatal and infancy home visiting by nurses: from randomized trials to community replication. *Prev Sci.* 2002;3(3):153-172.

Pears KC, Fisher PA, Heywood CV, Bronz KD. Promoting school readiness in foster children. In: Saracho ON, Spodek B, eds. *Contemporary Perspectives on Social Learning in Early Childhood Education.* Charlotte, NC: Information Age Publishing; 2007:173-198.

Pears KC, Fisher PA, Kim HK, Bruce J, Healey CV, Yoerger K. Immediate effects of a school readiness intervention for children in foster care. *Early Educ Dev.* 2013;24(6):771-791.

Pears KC, Kim HK, Fisher PA. Effects of a school readiness intervention for children in foster care on oppositional and aggressive behaviors in kindergarten. *Child Youth Serv Rev.* 2012;34(12):2361-2366.

Reid JB, Eddy JM, Fetrow RA, Stoolmiller M. Description and immediate impacts of a preventive intervention for conduct problems. *Am J Community Psychol.* 1999;27(4):483-517.

Shaw DS, Dishion TJ, Supplee L, Gardner F, Arnds K. Randomized trial of a family-centered approach to the prevention of early conduct problems: 2-year effects of the family check-up in early childhood. *J Consult Clin Psychol.* 2006;74(1):1-9.

Smolkowski K, Biglan A, Barrera M, Taylor T, Black C, Blair J. Schools and Homes in Partnership (SHIP): long-term effects of a preventive intervention focused on social behavior and reading skill in early elementary school. *Prev Sci.* 2005;6(2):113-125.

Snyder FJ, Vuchinich S, Acock A, et al. Impact of the Positive Action program on school-level indicators of academic achievement, absenteeism, and disciplinary outcomes: a matched-pair, cluster randomized, controlled trial. *J Res Educ Eff.* 2010;3(1):26-55.

Tolan P, Gorman-Smith D, Henry D. Supporting families in a high-risk setting: proximal effects of the SAFEChildren preventive intervention. *J Consult Clin Psychol.* 2004;72(5):855-869.

Tolan PH, Gorman-Smith D, Henry D, Schoeny M. The benefits of booster interventions: evidence from a family-focused prevention program. *Prev Sci.* 2009;10(4): 287-297.

Wang Y, Storr CL, Green KM, et al. The effect of two elementary school-based prevention interventions on being offered tobacco and the transition to smoking. *Drug and Alcohol Depend.* 2012;120(1–3):202-208.

Webster-Stratton C, Reid MJ, Hammond M. Treating children with early-onset conduct problems: intervention outcomes for parent, child, and teacher training. *J Clin Child Adolesc Psychol.* 2004;33(1):105-124.

Webster-Stratton C, Reid MJ, Stoolmiller M. Preventing conduct problems and improving school readiness: evaluation of the Incredible Years Teacher and Child Training Programs in high-risk schools. *J Child Psychol Psychiatry.* 2008;49(5):471-488.

Webster-Stratton C, Reid MJ. The Incredible Years Parents, Teachers and Children Training Series: a multifaceted treatment approach for young children with conduct problems. In: Kazdin AE, Weisz JR, eds. *Evidence-Based Psychotherapies for Children and Adolescents.* 2nd ed. New York, NY: Guilford Publications; 2010.

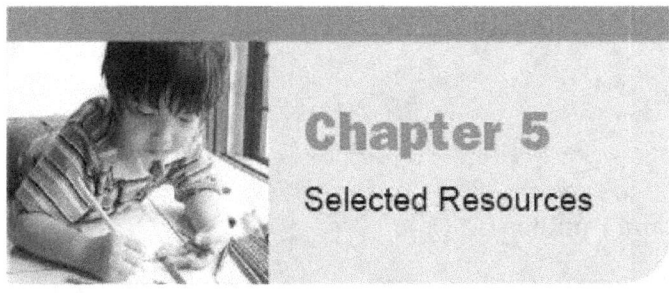

## Chapter 5
### Selected Resources

Below are resources relevant to drug abuse prevention. Information on NIDA's website is followed by websites for other federal agencies and other public and private organizations. These resources are excellent sources of information on research-based early childhood drug prevention programs.

**National Institute on Drug Abuse (NIDA)**
**National Institutes of Health (NIH)**
**U.S. Department of Health and Human Services (HHS)**

NIDA's website (www.drugabuse.gov) provides factual information on all aspects of drug abuse, particularly the effects of drugs on the brain and body, the prevention of drug abuse among children and adolescents, the latest research on treatment for addiction, and statistics on the extent of drug abuse in the United States. The website allows visitors to access publications, public service announcements and posters, science education curricula, research reports and fact sheets on specific drugs or classes of drugs, and the *NIDA NOTES* newsletter. The site also links to related websites in the public and private sectors.

The Prevention Research Branch (PRB) of NIDA's Division of Epidemiology, Services and Prevention Research (DESPR) website is a great resource for more information on the latest research on the prevention of drug abuse.

**Other Federal Resources**

**U.S. Department of Education (ED)**
400 Maryland Avenue, SW
Washington, DC 20202
Phone: 800-872-5327
www.ed.gov

> **Office of Safe and Healthy Students** (in the Office of Elementary and Secondary Education (OESE)) http://www2.ed.gov/about/offices/list/oese/oshs/index.html

**U.S. Department of Health and Human Services (HHS)**
200 Independence Avenue, SW
Washington, DC 20201
Phone: 877-696-6775
www.hhs.gov

### Administration for Children and Families (ACF)
370 L'Enfant Promenade, SW
Washington, DC 20447
Phone: 202-401-9200
www.acf.hhs.gov
> Children's Bureau www.acf.hhs.gov/programs/cb
> Office of Child Care (OCC) www.acf.hhs.gov/programs/occ
> Office of Head Start (OHS) www.acf.hhs.gov/programs/ohs
> Office of Planning, Research and Evaluation (OPRE)
> www.acf.hhs.gov/programs/opre

### Administration for Community Living (ACL)
One Massachusetts Avenue, NW
Washington, DC 20001
Phone: 202-401-4634
Administration on Intellectual and Developmental Disabilities (AIDD)
www.acl.gov/programs/aidd/index.aspx

### Centers for Disease Control and Prevention (CDC)
1600 Clifton Road
Atlanta, GA 30329
Phone: 800-CDC-INFO (800-232-4636)
www.cdc.gov
> National Center for Chronic Disease Prevention and Health Promotion
> (NCCDPHP) www.cdc.gov/chronicdisease/index.htm
> Division of Violence Prevention (DVP) www.cdc.gov/violenceprevention/
> > Child Maltreatment
> > www.cdc.gov/ViolencePrevention/childmaltreatment/index.html
> National Center on Birth Defects and Developmental Disabilities (NCBDDD)
> www.cdc.gov/ncbddd/index.html
> > Child Development
> > www.cdc.gov/ncbddd/childdevelopment/index.html
> > *Legacy for Children*™
> > www.cdc.gov/ncbddd/childdevelopment/legacy.html
> > Learn the Signs. Act Early. www.cdc.gov/ncbddd/actearly/
> > Parent Information www.cdc.gov/parents/index.html
> National Center for Injury Prevention and Control (NCIPC)
> www.cdc.gov/injury
> > *Protect the Ones you Love: Child Injuries are Preventable*
> > www.cdc.gov/safechild/

**Health Resources and Services Administration (HRSA)**
5600 Fishers Lane
Rockville, MD 20857
Phone: 888-ASK-HRSA (888-275-4772)
www.hrsa.gov
>   Maternal and Child Health Bureau (MCHB) www.mchb.hrsa.gov

**Indian Health Service (IHS)**
The Reyes Building
801 Thompson Avenue
Rockville, MD 20852
Phone: 301-443-3593
www.ihs.gov

**National Institutes of Health (NIH)**
9000 Rockville Pike
Bethesda, MD 20892
Phone: 301-496-4000
www.nih.gov

>   **The Eunice Kennedy Shriver National Institute of Child Health and Human Development (NICHD)**
>   Bldg 31, Room 2A32, MSC 2425
>   31 Center Drive
>   Bethesda, MD 20892-2425
>   Phone: 800-370-2943
>   www.nichd.nih.gov

>   **National Institute on Alcohol Abuse and Alcoholism (NIAAA)**
>   5635 Fishers Lane, MSC 9304
>   Bethesda, MD 20892-9304
>   Phone: 301-443-3860
>   www.niaaa.nih.gov

>   **National Institute of Environmental Health Sciences (NIEHS)**
>   111 T.W. Alexander Drive
>   Research Triangle Park, NC 27709
>   Phone: 919-541-3345
>   www.niehs.nih.gov
>>   Children's Health
>>   www.niehs.nih.gov/health/topics/population/children/index.cfm
>>   Environmental Health Topics
>>   www.niehs.nih.gov/health/topics/index.cfm

**National Institute of Mental Health (NIMH)**
6001 Executive Boulevard, Room 6200, MSC 9663
Bethesda, MD 20892-9663
Phone: 866-615-6464
www.nimh.nih.gov

**National Library of Medicine (NLM)**
8600 Rockville Pike
Bethesda, MD 20894
Phone: 888-FIND-NLM (888-346-3656)
www.nlm.nih.gov

**Office of the Assistant Secretary for Planning and Evaluation (ASPE)**
200 Independence Avenue, SW
Washington, DC 20201
Phone: 877-696-6775
www.aspe.hhs.gov
Early Childhood and School Readiness
http://aspe.hhs.gov/office_specific/topic3.cfm?tpcid=51&topic=Early%20Childhoo
d%20and%20School%20Readiness&office=HSP&CFID=379200&CFTOKEN=80912
328

**Substance Abuse and Mental Health Services Administration (SAMHSA)**
1 Choke Cherry Road
Rockville, Maryland 20857
Phone: 877-SAMHSA-7 (877-726-4727)
www.samhsa.gov
      Center for Substance Abuse Prevention (CSAP) www.samhsa.gov/prevention

**U.S. Department of Agriculture**
1400 Independence Avenue, SW
Washington, DC 20250
Phone: 202-720-2791
www.usda.gov
      National Institute of Food and Agriculture (NIFA) www.csrees.usda.gov

**Office of National Drug Control Policy (ONDCP)**
P.O. Box 6000
Rockville, MD 20849
Phone: 800-666-3332
www.whitehouse.gov/ondcp

## Other Selected Resources

### Academic Professional Organizations

**American Academy of Child and Adolescent Psychiatry (AACAP)**
3615 Wisconsin Avenue, NW
Washington, DC 20016
Phone: 202-966-7300
www.aacap.org

**American Academy of Family Physicians (AAFP)**
11400 Tomahawk Creek Parkway
Leawood, KS 66211
Phone: 913-906-6000
www.aafp.org
www.familydoctor.org

**American Academy of Pediatrics (AAP)**
141 Northwest Point Boulevard
Elk Grove Village, IL 60007
Phone: 800-433-9016
www.aap.org

**American Psychological Association (APA)**
750 First Street, NE
Washington, DC 20002
Phone: 800-374-2121
www.apa.org

**American Society of Addiction Medicine (ASAM)**
4601 North Park Avenue
Upper Arcade, Suite 101
Chevy Chase, MD 20815
Phone: 301-656-3920
www.asam.org

**International Society on Infant Studies (ISIS)**
350 Main Street
Malden, MA 02148
Phone: 800-835-6770
www.isisweb.org

**National Association for the Education Young Children (NAEYC)**
1313 L Street, NW
Suite 500
Washington, DC 20005
Phone: 800-424-2460
www.naeyc.org

**National Association of Pediatric Nurse Practitioners (NAPNAP)**
5 Hanover Square
Suite 1401
New York, NY 10004
Phone: 917-746-8300
www.napnap.org

**National Association of School Nurses**
1100 Wayne Avenue
Suite 925
Silver Spring, MD 20910
Phone: 240-821-1130
www.nasn.org

**National Council on Family Relations (NCFR)**
1201 West River Parkway
Suite 200
Minneapolis, MN 55454
Phone: 888-781-9331
www.ncfr.org

**National Hispanic Science Network (NHSN)**
Health Sciences Center, New Orleans
Louisiana State University
1901 Perdido Street
New Orleans, LA 70112
Phone: 504-568-6187
http://nhsn.med.miami.edu

**Society of Pediatric Nurses (SPN)**
330 North Wabash Avenue
Suite 2000
Chicago, IL 60611
Phone: 312-321-5154
www.pedsnurses.org

**Society for Prevention Research (SPR)**
11240 Waples Mill Road
Suite 200
Fairfax, VA 22030
Phone: 703-934-4850
www.preventionresearch.org

**Society for Research in Child Development (SRCD)**
2950 South State Street
Suite 401
Ann Arbor, MI 48104
Phone: 734-926-0600
www.srcd.org

**Other Non-Governmental Resources**
**Annie E. Casey Foundation**
701 St. Paul Street
Baltimore, MD 21202
Phone: 410-547-6600
www.aecf.org

**Center for the Study and Prevention of Violence (CSPV)**
Institute of Behavioral Science
University of Colorado Boulder
483 UCB
Boulder, CO 80309-0483
Phone: 303-492-1032
www.colorado.edu/cspv/blueprints/

**Casey Family Programs**
2001 Eighth Avenue
Suite 2700
Seattle, WA 98121
Phone: 206-282-7300
www.casey.org

**Collaborative for Academic, Social, and Emotional Learning (CASEL)**
815 West Van Buren Street
Suite 210
Chicago, IL 60607
Phone: 312-226-3770
www.casel.org

**CASAColumbia**
633 Third Avenue, 19th Floor
New York, NY 10017
Phone: 212-841-5200
www.casacolumbia.org

**Children's Defense Fund**
25 E Street, NW
Washington, DC 20001
Phone: 800-CDF-1200 (800-233-1200)
www.childrensdefense.org

**Community Anti-Drug Coalitions of America (CADCA)**
625 Slaters Lane
Suite 300
Alexandria, VA 22314
Phone: 800-54-CADCA (800-542-2322)
www.cadca.org

**Drug Strategies, Inc.**
1150 Connecticut Avenue, NW, Suite 800
Washington, DC 20036
Phone: 202-289-9070
www.drugstrategies.org

**Foundation for Child Development**
295 Madison Avenue
40th Floor
New York, NY 10017
Phone: 212-867-5777
www.fcd-us.org

**Mentor Foundation USA**
2900 K Street NW, South Building
Washington, DC 20007
Phone: 202-536-1594
www.mentorfoundation.org/usa

**National Asian Pacific American Families Against Substance Abuse (NAPAFASA)**
340 East 2nd Street
Suite 409
Los Angeles, CA 90012
Phone: 213-625-5795
www.napafasa.org

**National Black Child Development Institute (NBCDI)**
1313 L Street, NW
Suite 110
Washington, DC 20005
Phone: 800-556-2234
202-833-2220
www.nbcdi.org

**National Head Start Association (NHSA)**
1651 Prince Street
Alexandria, VA 22314
Phone: 866-677-8724
703-739-0875
www.nhsa.org

**Partnership for Drug-Free Kids**
352 Park Avenue South
9th Floor
New York, NY 10010
Phone: 212-922-1560
www.drugfree.org

**Robert Wood Johnson Foundation**
Route 1 and College Road East
P.O. Box 2316
Princeton, NJ 08543
Phone: 877-843-7953
www.rwjf.org

**Frank Porter Graham Child Development Institute**
University of North Carolina at Chapel Hill
CB 8180
Chapel Hill, NC 27599
Phone: 919-966-2622
www.fpg.unc.edu

**WilliamT. Grant Foundation**
570 Lexington Avenue
18th Floor
New York, NY 10022
Phone: 212-752-0071
www.wtgrantfoundation.org

**Zero to Three: National Center for Infants, Toddlers, and Families**
1255 23rd Street, NW
Suite 350
Washington, DC 20037
Phone: 202-638-1144
www.zerotothree.org

**Other Resources**

**National Prevention Network (NPN)**
National Association of State Alcohol/Drug Abuse Directors (NASADAD)
1025 Connecticut Avenue, NW
Suite 605
Washington, DC 20036
Phone: 202-293-0090
www.nasadad.org/national-prevention-network

**United Nations Office on Drugs and Crime (UNODC)**
Vienna International Centre
Wagramer Strasse 5
A 1400 Vienna
Austria
Phone: +(43) (1) 26060
http://www.unodc.org/

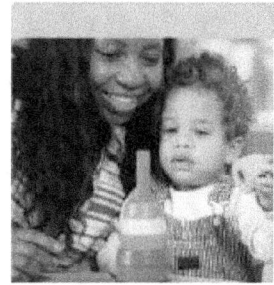

# Appendix 1

## From Theory To Outcomes—Designing Evidence-Based Interventions

Through theory, observation, and behavioral study, scientists have determined that select facets of human behavior can be changed over time. Specifically, the effects of malleable risk factors can be reduced, protective factors can be enhanced or developed, and resources can be accessed. An important avenue for accomplishing this is through prevention interventions that develop knowledge, skills, and competencies in the targeted individual(s). This provides the basic rationale for the conception and design of prevention intervention programs.

### From Theory to Intervention

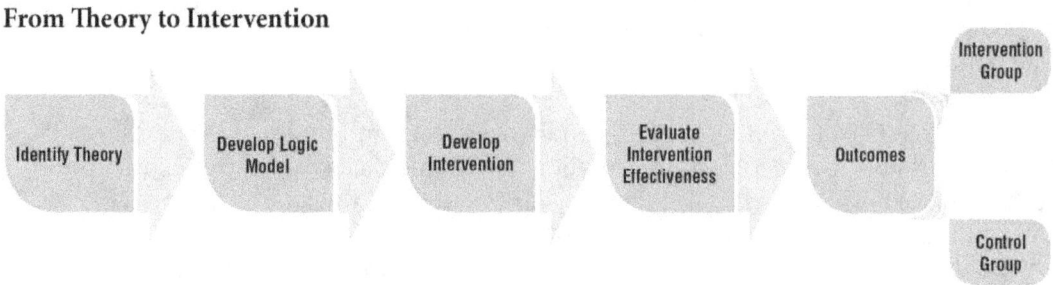

Design of science-based interventions begins at the theoretical level, with:

- *Developmental theories* that explain human growth and maturation; the normal course of physical, psychological, emotional, and cognitive changes; and what motivates humans to behave in particular ways
- *Ecological theories* that specify the contexts within which individuals develop and function and strive to explain the factors within contexts that influence changes in behavior
- *Cognitive theories* that focus on internal states such as motivation, problem-solving, decision-making, and attention
- *Behavior analytic theories* that focus on how behaviors and habits are acquired and can be changed

These theories help researchers think about how patterns of behaviors develop, what motivates individuals to behave in specific ways, and what risk and protective factors should be examined. The influence of theory can be traced throughout the processes of conceptualizing, developing, and testing an intervention. Theory informs thinking about what internal and contextual factors and processes may be modifiable; this information is then used in the development of the *logic model*.

Logic models graphically explain how changes in malleable risk and protective factors and behaviors will take place over time to produce positive outcomes. From the logic model described in "Intervening in Early Childhood" (see "Logic Model for Intervening in Early Childhood to Prevent Drug Abuse"), an intervention is developed, including the specification of knowledge and activities designed to strengthen the resources and capacities identified as crucial to providing protection against and reducing risk factors and associated problem behaviors.

## Intervention Timing, Context, and Components

As discussed in "Why is Early Childhood Important to Substance Abuse Prevention?," life course transitions in childhood often signal new or evolving physical, cognitive, social, and emotional development and represent peak times of vulnerability to various risk factors. Prevention interventions are designed and tested for specific stages of development, with a focus on fostering optimal development as the child encounters new internal and external capacities, social relationships, and contexts. For instance, the expectations for performance associated with new phases of life can trigger anxiety and self-doubt among many children. Providing experiences with and practice in negotiating new situations during these transitions can foster confidence and competence, thereby maximizing the potential for optimal development.

As was described in "Intervening in Early Childhood," interventions are generally targeted to the context that is most central to the target population—the proximal context. The most important context of very early development is the family, and thus this is the focus of prevention interventions for the prenatal through infancy and toddlerhood periods. Interventions may be delivered in the home or in other contexts with which families interact.** Other contexts, like school, become increasingly important for children at older ages.

Intervention components specify what knowledge, skills, and competencies are addressed in an intervention to achieve the target outcome. Components are specific to target populations and, within an intervention, multiple actors may be defined as target populations. For example, family-based programs often include parent and child behavioral outcomes and classroom interventions often include both teacher and child outcomes. Moreover, interventions that combine contexts—such as family and school—could target the child, the caregivers, and the teachers. Thus, the targeted knowledge, skills, and competencies would be specific to those intervention populations and can be very precisely defined.

---

** This is the case with two examples of the NIDA-supported interventions for children under the age of 3. The Nurse Family Partnership intervention (www.nursefamilypartnership.org) sends nurses to the home to train young mothers and can take advantage of the public health system for implementation. The Early Steps intervention screens for mothers in need of services through an existing program for at-risk families called Women, Infants, and Children (WIC), who are then visited, usually in the home, by a trained clinician. Together they decide what resources and services would be most helpful for the child and family.

The diagram "How Interventions Work" illustrates several key features that help in understanding how interventions work. *Moderators* are aspects of the people who are targeted by the intervention and influence the intervention's design and outcomes but cannot be changed—such as age, sex, race, and socio-economic factors such as poverty. *Modifiable risk factors* are the knowledge, behaviors, attitudes, intentions, skills, and competencies that the intervention attempts to change. The intervention often includes:

- activities designed to promote skill development in specific areas such as parenting
- environmental change strategies, such as modifying classroom management style to reduce the aggressive behaviors of some children
- provision of services to help in the development of specific competencies such as academic skills through tutoring
- community-level change strategies such as changing minors' access to alcohol or tobacco through policy enforcement

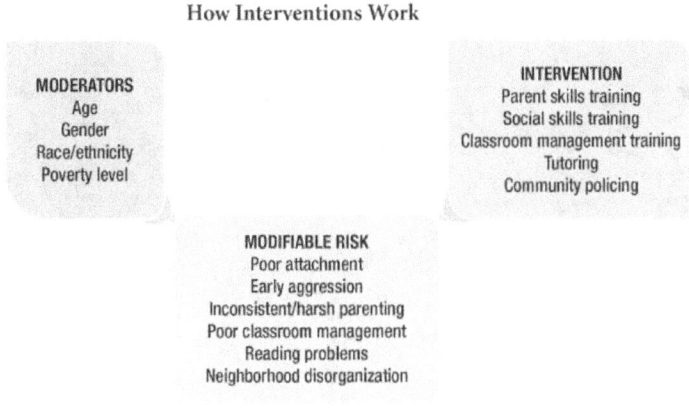

How Interventions Work

## Program Evaluation and Assessment of Benefit-Cost

Prevention interventions developed using scientific methods go through these stages of theory and logic model conceptualization. In addition, they are subjected to testing, usually in a randomized controlled trial (RCT) or other rigorous research design. An RCT randomly assigns participants to intervention and control conditions. The advantage of this method and other rigorous research designs is that they make it possible to draw conclusions about the effectiveness of an intervention without being concerned that the outcomes are related to some other population or contextual factor that was not taken into account.

Through the evaluation and comparison of measures of current status among intervention and control group participants at multiple time points before, during, and after the intervention, changes in behaviors, attitudes, intentions, skills, and knowledge can be assessed to determine if the expected positive results were achieved.

Continued assessment of intervention-group children and families and comparison with control-group families into adolescence—and in some cases, into early adulthood and beyond—allows researchers to draw conclusions about the impact of intervening in early childhood on outcomes across the course of development, including effects on the initiation or reduction of drug use and related problems. Long-term follow-up of study participants informs understanding of program effects and provides information that can be used to determine the benefits of early interventions relative to their costs. Some of the existing research has not yet been able to follow participants to the point at which drug use, abuse, and addiction occur; for such programs, the assessment of benefit-cost must be estimated. Participants in other programs have been followed into adolescence and young adulthood, and researchers have been able to directly measure outcomes such as drug involvement, educational attainment, criminality, mental health problems, and health-risking sexual behaviors. When this is the case, a direct comparison of those who received an intervention versus those who did not receive it can determine the benefit-cost of the program in preventing negative and promoting positive outcomes (see "Benefit–Cost Examples for Early Childhood Programs").

---

**Benefit–Cost Examples for Early Childhood Programs**

Research on the benefits relative to costs of early childhood prevention interventions has shown positive results. Some examples of benefit-cost data of interventions with long-term follow-up data are:

- Durham Connects—$3.02 saved for each dollar invested (Dodge et al., 2013b)
- Nurse Family Partnership—$2.88 saved for each dollar invested (Aos et al., 2004)
- Seattle Social Development Project—$3.14 saved for each dollar invested (Aos et al., 2004)
- Good Behavior Game (used in the Classroom-Centered Intervention)—$25.92 saved for each dollar invested (Aos et al., 2004)

Other programs with long-term follow-up data have not shown benefits this dramatic. However, the listed examples point out the extent to which a well-conceptualized and implemented intervention for very young children can benefit society tangibly, not to mention the improved quality of life for children and families that comes from preventing substance abuse and other problems. The tables below indicate which of the early interventions included in this review have economic analysis information (e.g., cost, benefit-cost, or cost effectiveness analysis).

---

## Infancy and Toddlerhood

| Program | Economic Analysis Information |
|---|---|
| **Durham Connects** | Cost of the intervention; benefit-cost analysis; Emergency health care service savings (Dodge et al., 2013b) |
| **Early Steps, Family Check Up** | N/A |
| **Family Spirit** | N/A |
| **Nurse Family Partnership** | Savings in government spending (Olds et al., 2010) Benefit-cost analysis (Karolyv et al., 2005; Aos et al., 2004) |

## Preschool

| Program | Economic Analysis Information |
| --- | --- |
| **Incredible Years-Spirit** | N/A |
| **Multidimensional Treatment Foster Care for Preschoolers** | N/A |

## Transition to Elementary School

| Program | Economic Analysis Information Available? |
| --- | --- |
| **Caring School Community Program** | N/A |
| **Classroom-Centered Intervention (Good Behavior Game)** | Benefit-cost analysis (Aos et al., 2004; Miller & Hendrie, 2008) |
| **Linking the Interests of Families and Teachers** | N/A |
| **Raising Healthy Children** | N/A |
| **SAFEChildren** | Cost of program(National Registry: SAFEChildren, 2014) |
| **Seattle Social Development Program** | Benefit-cost analysis(Aos et al., 2004; Miller & Hendrie, 2008) |
| **Early Risers "Skills for Success" Risk Prevention Program** | Cost of program(National Registry: Early Risers, 2014) |
| **Kids in Transition to School** | N/A |
| **Fast Track Trial for Conduct Problems** | Cost of conduct problems (Foster & Jones, 2005) Cost effectiveness analysis (Foster et al., 2006) |
| **Incredible Years** | Cost effectiveness analysis (Foster et al., 2007) |
| **Positive Action** | Cost of program(National Registry: Positive Action, 2014) |
| **Schools and Homes in Partnership** | N/A |

## Selected References

Aos S, Lieb R, Mayfield J, Miller M, Pennucci A. Benefits and costs of prevention and early intervention programs for youth. Olympia, WA: Washington State Institute for Public Policy; 2004. Document No. 04-07-3901. http://www.wsipp.wa.gov/ReportFile/881/Wsipp_Benefits-and-Costs-of-Prevention-and-Early-Intervention-Programs-for-Youth_Summary-Report.pdf. Published September 17, 2004. Accessed February 3, 2015.

Dodge KA, Goodman WB, Murphy RA, O'Donnell K, Sato J. Randomized controlled trial evaluation of universal postnatal nurse home visiting: impacts on child emergency medical care at age 12-months. *Pediatrics.* 2013;132:S140-S146.

Foster EM, Jones DE. The high costs of aggression: public expenditures resulting from conduct disorder. *Am J Public Health.* 2005;95(10):1767-1772.

Foster EM, Jones D, Conduct Problems Prevention Research Group. Can a costly intervention be cost-effective? An analysis of violence prevention. *Arch Gen Psychiatry.* 2006;63(11):1284-1291.

Foster EM, Olchowski AE, Webster-Stratton CH. Is stacking intervention components cost-effective? An analysis of the Incredible Years program. *J Am Acad Child Adolesc Psychiatry.* 2007;46(11):1414-1424.

Karoly LA, Kilburn MR, Cannon J. *Early Childhood Interventions: Proven Results, Future Promise.* Santa Monica, CA: RAND Corporation; 2005.

Miller T, Hendrie D. *Substance Abuse Prevention Dollars and Cents: A Cost-Benefit Analysis.* Rockville, MD: Center for Substance Abuse Prevention, Substance Abuse and Mental Health Services Administration; 2008. HHS Pub. No. (SMA) 07-4298. http://store.samhsa.gov/shin/content/SMA07-4298/SMA07-4298.pdf.

National Registry of Evidence-Based Programs and Practices. *Intervention Summary: SAFEChildren.* Rockville, MD: Substance Abuse and Mental Health Services Administration; 2014. http://nrepp.samhsa.gov/ViewIntervention.aspx?id=40. Reviewed: October 2007.

National Registry of Evidence-Based Programs and Practices. *Intervention Summary: Early Risers "Skills for Success."* Rockville, MD: Substance Abuse and Mental Health Services Administration; 2014. http://nrepp.samhsa.gov/ViewIntervention.aspx?id=304. Reviewed May 2007.

National Registry of Evidence-based Programs and Practices. *Intervention Summary: Positive Action.* Rockville, MD: Substance Abuse and Mental Health Services Administration; 2014. http://nrepp.samhsa.gov/ViewIntervention.aspx?id=78. Reviewed December 2006.

Olds DL, Kitzman H, Cole R, et al. Enduring effects of prenatal and infancy home visiting by nurses on maternal life course and government spending: follow-up of a randomized trial among children at age 12 years. *Arch Pediatr Adolesc Med.* 2010;164(5):419-424.

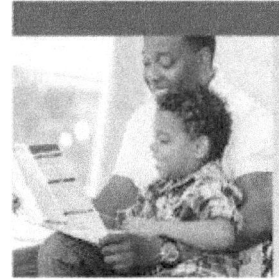

# Appendix 2
## Selecting and Implementing an Intervention

## Determining Community Risk and Protective Factors

Before selecting a prevention program or developing a comprehensive plan, it is important for communities to determine what risk factors may be contributing to problem behaviors and what resources the community has available to address the problem(s). Assessment of risk and protective factors is used to identify the problem(s) of interest through archival searches for information available in existing community databases (e.g., poverty level; access to nutritious food and health care; child accidents and maltreatment; abandoned/substandard housing; access to alcohol, tobacco, drugs, and firearms; toxic exposure) and through surveys of community members to assess family, school, and community functioning. Assessing these factors can help identify the most pressing problems facing a community. Community prevention leaders can then select the targeted problem to intervene upon (see "Examples of Community Risk Assessment").

### Examples of Community Risk Assessment

Below are two examples of risk and protective factor assessments at the school and community levels. The first example shows the results of surveying students within a high school about specific risk and protective factors. The resulting bar charts provide information on factors that can then be matched to specific evidence-based interventions.

In this particular example, community coalitions identified specific factors that needed to be reduced (risk factors; top graph) or increased (protective factors; bottom graph) and selected evidence-based prevention interventions to address them. The graphs illustrate how communities compare with the average for all schools within the school district and the national average on measures of protective factors at the community, family, school, and peer-individual levels. As shown in the top graph, for High School 'N,' ratings for several risk factors are significantly higher than those for other schools in the school district and the national average; the community selected one of these, "Favorable attitude toward drug use," as the risk factor they wanted to work on decreasing for this school (yellow arrow). As shown in the bottom graph, the value for the protective factor "Social skills" in High School 'N' was found to be a significantly lower compared to ratings for other schools in the school district and the national average, and the community selected this as the protective factor they wanted to work on increasing for that school (yellow arrow).

This framework could be adapted for use with early interventions. For example, data could include archival measures of public health data on prenatal visits by mothers, birth weights, social service records on child abuse and neglect, and access to local and county support services. Risk and protective factors could be determined through national data sets that provide information at the community level as well as by parent reports of child and family behaviors.

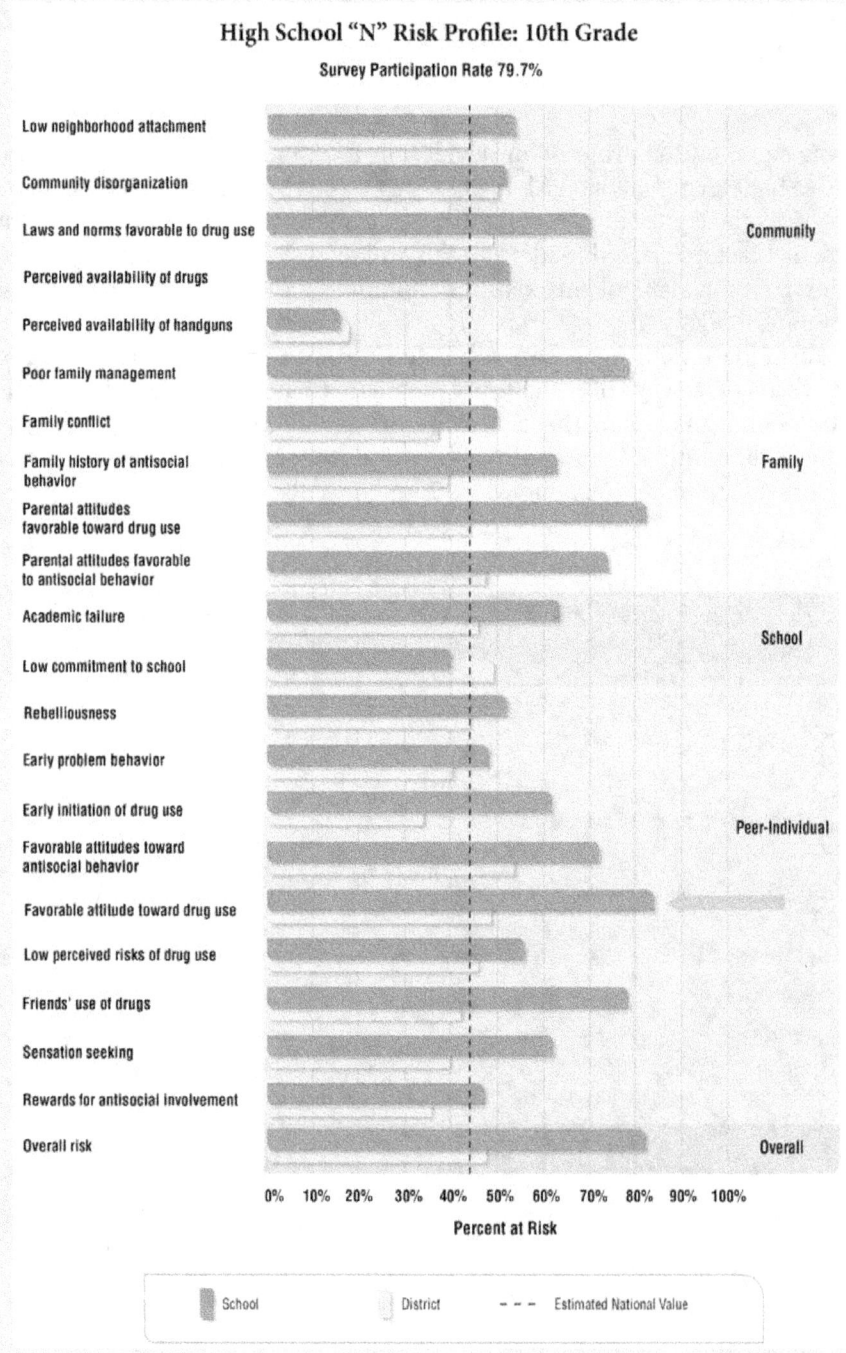

**High School "N" Risk Profile: 10th Grade**

Survey Participation Rate 79.7%

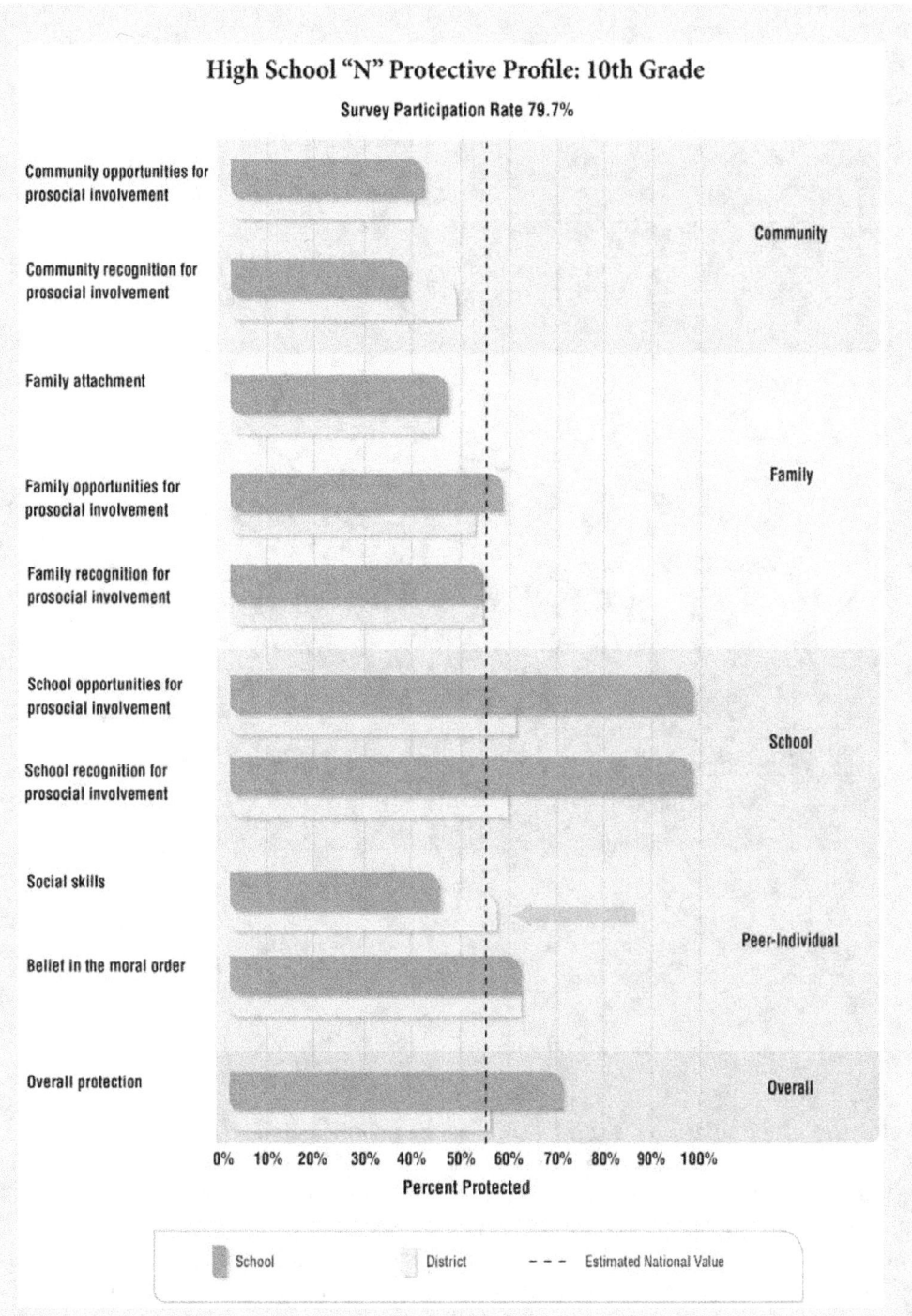

## High School "N" Protective Profile: 10th Grade

**Survey Participation Rate 79.7%**

Source: Hawkins, JD. Preventing Teen Smoking, Drinking and Violence Community Wide: Results from the Randomized Trial of Communities That Care. *Division of Epidemiology, Services and Prevention Research (DESPR) Seminar, National Institute on Drug Abuse, Rockville, MD; 2011.*

The second example provides a representation of substance abuse risk and protective
factors within a geographic community area. Based on youth surveys and community
records, 23 risk factors and 10 protective factors were examined in three neighborhoods of
a California community. The peaks within the three neighborhoods in the figure below
indicate elevated risk, with neighborhood #2 showing the highest elevation of risk factors.
Communities can use this information to decide where to implement evidence-based
substance abuse prevention interventions in order to address specific risk and protective
factors.

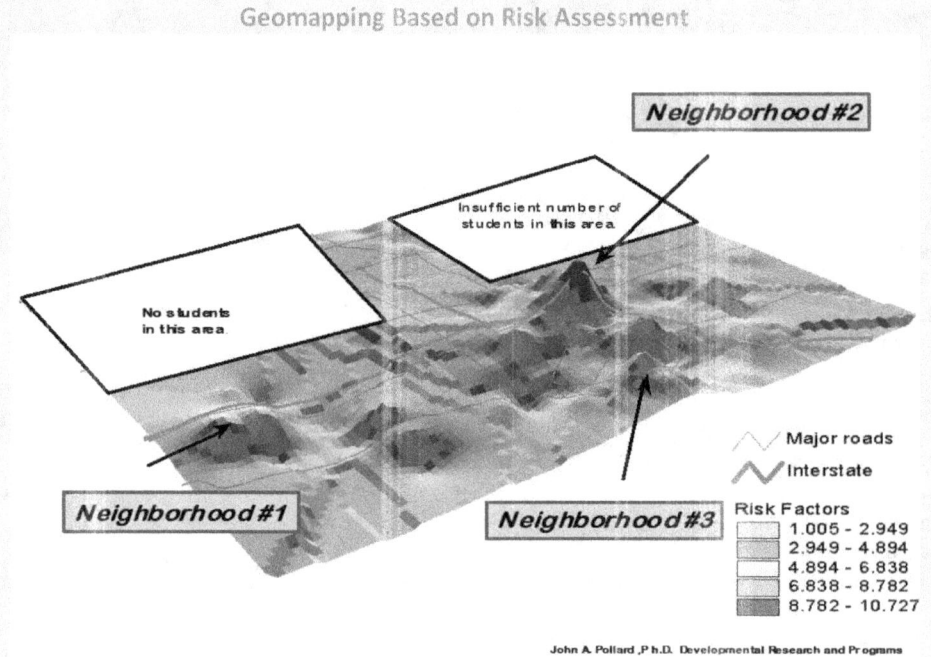

Geomapping Based on Risk Assessment

## Identifying the Target Population

Identifying the subpopulation most impacted by the problems isolated through the
community assessment of risk and protective factors will help determine the population to
be targeted for intervention. The target population is defined based on characteristics of
the individuals or group to be addressed by the intervention. For interventions addressing
childhood problems, age or developmental period is usually the most important defining
characteristic. Other characteristics to consider in defining the target populations include:
gender, race/ethnicity, health status, and socio-economic status. Another significant
defining characteristic of target populations is level of risk. Risk assessments help in
defining individuals and subpopulations at elevated risk due to internal, behavioral,
familial, and environmental factors.

## Adapting Programs

One question that is sometimes asked is whether childhood prevention interventions need to be modified for implementation with populations or contexts that differ from the original research. Unfortunately, this question has not been adequately addressed through research. Minor changes to original program materials to make the people, contexts, and examples more relevant to a specific group have been found to have little effect on intervention outcomes. Generally speaking, significant changes to the intervention structure and content are not recommended, as there is limited evidence on how these types of changes will affect outcomes. When a target population or context differs markedly from those targeted in available science-based interventions, a new intervention tailored to meet that population's specific needs (e.g., cultural or contextual needs) may need to be designed. An example of one such program, Family Spirit (described in "Research-Based Early Intervention Substance Abuse Prevention Programs") intervenes with very young poor mothers on American Indian reservations (Barlow et al., 2006).

Another adaptation that may need to be made is providing program support services to participants to make an intervention more accessible to them. Services may include transportation, care for other children in the family, snacks or meals, and compressed programming (e.g., offering fewer but longer sessions). Accommodations can lessen the burden associated with attending a program, help to build social support among members of the intervention group, and help keep participants coming to the program.

## Collecting Data

Collecting data before, during, and after the evidence-based intervention is implemented at the local level is important as it allows the implementer to assess whether the intervention is producing effects similar to those in the original research and, if not, to help in determining why. It helps community prevention leaders as they decide on next steps in maintaining the focus on the most important risk factors to address for developing a comprehensive prevention plan.

**Selected References**

Barlow A, Varipatis-Baker E, Speakman K, et al. 2006. Home-visiting intervention to improve child care among American Indian adolescent mothers: a randomized trial. *Arch Pediatr Adolesct Med.* 2006;160(11):1101-1107.

www.ingramcontent.com/pod-product-compliance
Lightning Source LLC
Chambersburg PA
CBHW082115220526
45472CB00009B/2188